UNDERSTANDING
COMPUTER RESOURCES
A HEALTHCARE PERSPECTIVE

UNDERSTANDING COMPUTER RESOURCES

A HEALTHCARE PERSPECTIVE

Stephen L. Priest

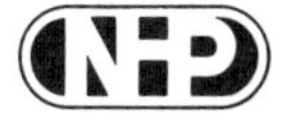

National Health Publishing
A Division of Williams & Wilkins

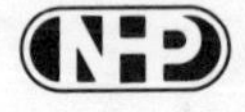

Published by
National Health Publishing
99 Painters Mill Road
Owings Mills, Maryland 21117
(301) 363-6400

A Division of Williams & Wilkins

Printed in the United States of America
First Printing

Designer: Sandy Renovetz
Compositor: National Health Publishing
Printer: Edwards Brothers

ISBN: 1-55857-012-8
LC: 88-063452

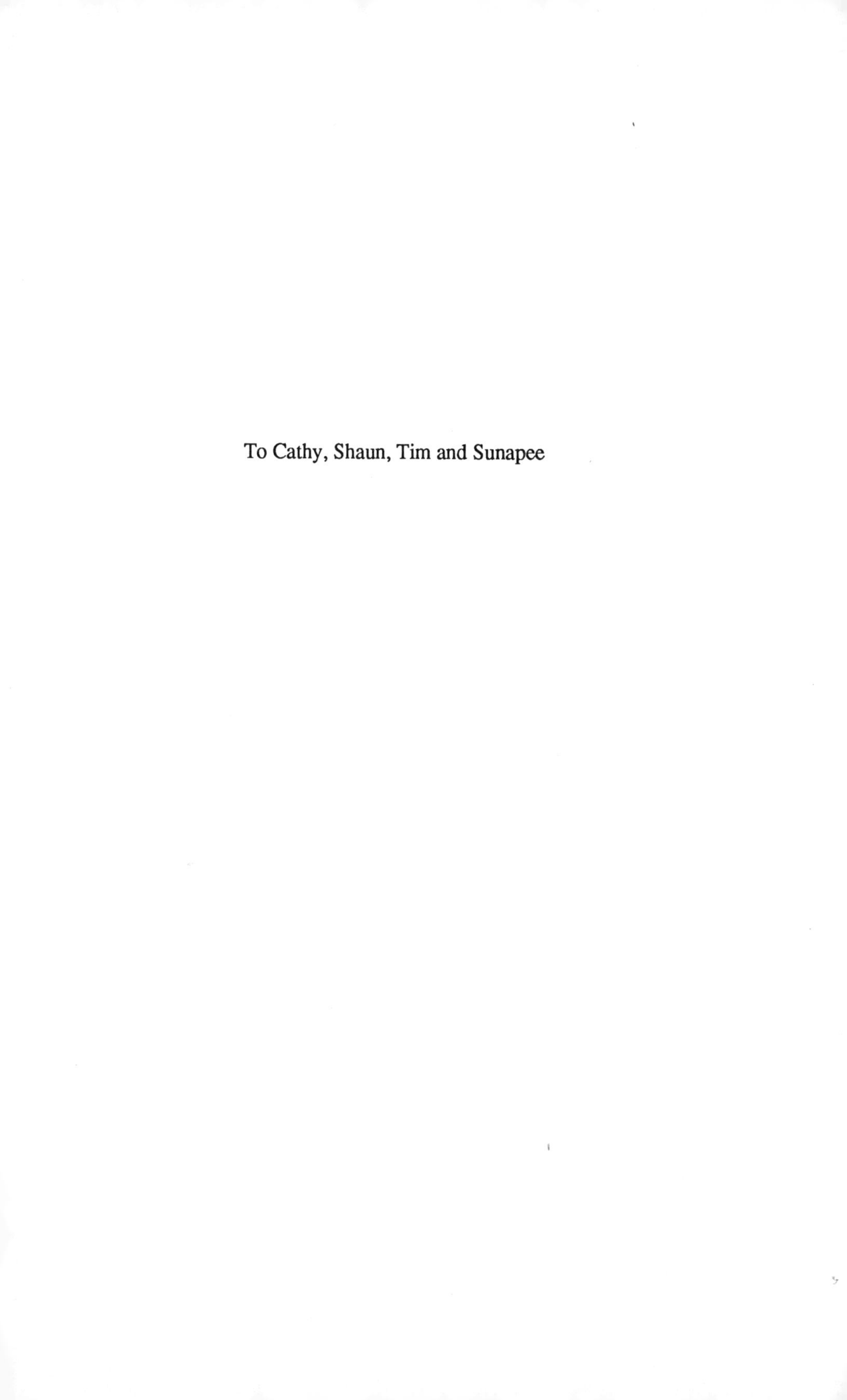

To Cathy, Shaun, Tim and Sunapee

CONTENTS

LIST OF FIGURES

LIST OF TABLES

FOREWORD

Whenever healthcare managers attempt to assess their computer resources, they frequently do so with considerable trepidation, in part because it is rarely the senior manager's area of professional expertise, and in part because too many senior managers have a less-than-global understanding of what constitutes "computer resources." Classroom instructors are regularly in search of clear and thoughtful approaches to enhance the education of current and prospective computer resource managers and users.

In *Understanding Computer Resources: A Healthcare Perspective,* Stephen L. Priest successfully handles the difficult task of providing a simple, well-organized and practical approach to this complex subject not only for the CEO, but for the end-user, the computer resource department, the consultant, and the instructor as well. "Success of the computer system," the author points out, "Comes when both users and computer resource professional staff understand each other's role and computer resource needs." Central to the text is the critical emphasis on the necessary interaction and communication between line managers and computer resource professionals. Indeed, not only the success of the computer system, but the success of the organizational system is heavily dependent upon this understanding.

All too frequently, computer resources are perceived in the same way that the three blind men described the elephant by touching different parts of the animal. The author offers a more global understanding for the reader in several ways. First, by clearly defining the respective roles of the computer resource players, and suggesting strategies for needs assessment, the book carefully sets the stage for the selection of appropriate resources (e.g., reporting formats to compare vendor responses to a RFP) and provides specific methods to define, select and implement computer hardware and software. Individual chapters address key decision points in the implementation "life cycle," computer resource monitoring techniques, when to centralize or decentralize computer resources, if and when consultants should be used, and guidelines for developing microcomputer policies. In addition to specific "how to" techniques, questions, and assignments both for the classroom and the operational setting on a variety of issues, mini-cases add insight to the enlarged potential for using computer resources. The author writes in a way which requires only a very basic level of understanding of computers. Throughout, the need for effective communication and interaction by all members of the organization is emphasized. This is particularly important in an industry where the environment is so dynamic. In a word, the author underscores the need for a "merge" of a different kind.

With each individual's medical record as the central focus of tomorrow's computer resource system—what Stephen Priest calls the "Healthcare Computer Network"—CEOs and planners of small and large healthcare provider systems of all kinds will gain some significant new insights. For example, managers of hospitals and of life care/assisted living/nursing home "campuses," will see the medical data matrix from a new perspective which emphasizes community linkages of many kinds.

Care is used to caution the reader about the risks associated with successful computer resource programs. For example, increased demand for computer services, when not managed properly can lead to costly and poor resource use. Fundamental planning, priority-setting and post implementation studies are essential ingredients in the long-term success of a thoughtful computer resource program.

Seasoned computer resource decision-makers, and classroom instructors, as well as those with limited experience will find the book a very valuable "computer resource."

Craig S. Higgins, Ph.D.
Chairman, Department of Health Care Administration
Stonehill College
North Easton, MA 02357

PREFACE

A number of books and articles discuss individual computer topics from the perspective of administration, the central computer resource (CR) management, or the end-user. Some books focus on the microcomputer and the many advances that it has made possible, and one senses that the microcomputer alone can serve the total organization. Other books address the value of an integrated computer system and how data can be shared among multiple users, avoiding duplicate entry and providing control of data. Microcomputers surely play a major role in today's organization, but senior management also needs management reports using data stored in more than one department. Few books combine and blend these topics—individual department roles using microcomputers and organization-wide mainframes and minicomputers—into a text that relates to senior management, the central CR management, and the end-user. This is the ambitious intent of this book. I hope to get senior management, central CR management, and the end-user to recognize each other's concerns and needs in the development and use of computer resources and services.

Microcomputers offer to individuals and organizations functions not available on centrally managed computers. The early 1980s witnessed a rapid growth in the number of people in various noncomputer vocations becoming familiar with microcomputer hardware, software, and application concepts. Today, professionals in administration, home care, physician office practice, nursing homes, public relations, mental health, finance, human resources, and various other support and ancillary areas require managers and staff to have an understanding of the capabilities of computer resources. This book provides those people with a perspective on the responsibilities and strategies for planning, managing, and monitoring computer resources. This objective builds on prior knowledge by providing the reader with sufficient strategies both to meet individual computer needs successfully by themselves and to use and work effectively with CR professionals.

The text has a minimal amount of computer jargon. It presents, by situation, the CR responsibilities of the people using the computer resources: senior management needing internal and external perspectives for such concerns as marketing, decision-making, planning, budgeting; the central computer manager trying to maximize the usage of automation while attempting to maintain control of its growth; and the user computer manager, the person in the user department responsible for meeting the department's objectives with the computer as its tool. The book can be used by students and practicing health-care professionals to prepare and visualize through case study their computer resource responsibilities, policies, and procedures.

Any manager, planner, or professional whose job is affected or will be changed by the use of computer resources should understand the concepts presented in this text and the vital role played by people in the successes and failures of computer resources and services. The underlying theme of the text is this: a computer system is successful when both users and CR professional staff understand each other's role and CR needs. Managers must recognize that successful computer systems require team efforts. This effort applies to the microcomputer user, and applies to the centrally managed mainframe and minicomputers.

The term "computer resources" is defined as those services, staff, and equipment that provide for automated information needs. These include microcomputers, minicomputers, mainframe computers, software applications, programmers, systems analysts, telecommunications, information centers, database administrators, office automation, printers, video display terminals, etc. These resources can be provided through a central CR staff and through a user area with independent CR management.

At one time, computers and formatted information were needed only by a few persons with the same information needs. Now there are computer system applications for every health-care vocation and every level of operation. As health-care information needs change and computer hardware and software make rapid technological advances, the roles of the people responsible for the growth and use of computer resources also change. The concerns of these managers are described in minicases throughout the book.

Computer resource concepts and concerns are applicable both to organizations with a central CR staff and to those that use outside CR vendors. They are applicable to an individual user area that has sole control over its computer resources. Indeed, many organizations use a combination of in-house, outside vendor, and user area services. It is important that organizations recognize the need to understand, manage, and control the current and future growth of their computer resources.

This book discusses areas that general management, central CR personnel, and end-users of computer systems must consider when beginning, managing, or expanding services. It attempts to explain from a user's and a central CR manager's perspective the management and operational requirements of the computer resources within the organizational structure.

For many years, data processing (DP) was considered a minor service, usually buried within the confines of the financial chain-of-command and tolerated for the sole purpose of offering clerical replacement services. Users often felt that they could obtain only those narrow services that DP could provide. Today's computer technology provides to every user area alternatives of obtaining CR services through the traditional centralized avenue, through the acquisition of microcomputers, or directly from CR vendors.

The computer resources responsibility currently enjoys senior status on organization charts. Almost all organizations now recognize the value of CR services and the value of the information provided to managers through those services. In fact, the need for and value of information have resulted in a call from all divisions of the organization to have CR systems and services immediately accessible.

Many ideas discussed in this text were refined in courses taught at Stonehill College (Easton, MA). These courses were offered to students in health-care administration, nursing, and business majors. In these courses, I blend my experience in establishing and maintaining computer resources with current literature on the topic. The primary emphasis is on real-life situations, both positive and negative, combined with textbook theory. Case study discussions are used extensively in an effort to apply principles to realistic situations.

Chapter 1 of the text presents some basic definitions and concepts. It defines an organization's computer resources. Topics discussed include the history of CRs and the position of central CR services in the organization. This chapter begins a discussion of the importance of senior management requiring and encouraging strong interaction between end-users and CR specialists.

Chapter 2 discusses the roles of the user computer resources manager (UCRM), the central computer resource manager (CCRM), and the steering committee. Chapter 3 is devoted entirely to the strategies that both users and computer resource staff use to ensure successful and effective computer systems and CR services. Computer implementation and management are no longer the concern of only a central CR staff. Users must participate in organization-wide CR decisions. CR management is also the responsibility of users.

Chapters 4 and 5 present various methods for quantitatively selecting microcomputer, minicomputer, and mainframe hardware and software. A method for the evaluation of an organization's and department's application and information needs is presented, with emphasis on my experiences.

Various examples are presented to show quantitative and subjective approaches and how they affect senior management, user, and central CR staff. Explained is the method used in putting together a request for proposal (RFP), including specific vendor response formats, and quantitatively analyzing vendor responses.

Chapter 6 presents the computer system life cycle and its role in implementing computer systems. This chapter relates the importance and concepts of systems analysis, user groups, training, implementation, combating computer viruses, and ongoing enhancements.

Chapter 7 discusses both the centralized and the distributed approaches to the use and control of computer resources. It offers a framework to explain how the management, systems development, computer operation, and database resources decision can be considered on a user area by user area basis. It addresses the usage of microcomputers on both an organizational and an individual area basis. It addresses choices of office automation from both the central perspective and that of the end-user.

Chapter 8 covers project priorities, follow-up cost/benefit analysis, long-range planning, and critical success factors to monitor CR satisfaction and costs. The need for formal methods to select and rank projects is emphasized, as is the importance of follow-up performance evaluations in ensuring the proper allocation of computer resources. Are the users of the CR services being satisfied? Are CR costs reasonable? These questions and others concerning computer resource management are addressed.

Chapter 9 uses many of the principles discussed in Chapters 1 through 8 and presents a diary of how one organization defined, selected, implemented, and managed an integrated computer resource. It presents the impact of the CR on various users and discusses how the success of the system can be attributed to the staff responsible for maintaining the resources. Chapter 10 describes a microcomputer policy. It is meant as an example to demonstrate the concepts discussed in the previous chapters.

Chapter 11 describes my perception of tomorrow's health-care computer resources as they will impact on hospitals, physicians' offices, home health agencies, satellite clinics, and nursing homes. It discusses a computer network where the individual's medical data is the focal point of the system, regardless of where the individual physically resides. Each chapter is followed by assignments intended to create dialogue and discussion.

The appendix is a real-life scenario of a private physician's office staffed by people who did not know and follow proper microcomputer usage procedures. Only after the entire patient database was nearly destroyed was attention paid to the risk of computer storage with proper backup and training.

ACKNOWLEDGMENTS

To attempt to name those people who have contributed to my understanding of computer resources would be impossible as I owe such a debt of gratitude to the many who have shared their ideas, opinions, facilities, and time with me. Be assured that the many examples and ideas expressed in this text are but a reflection of the people with whom I have been so fortunate to work.

Through coauthors of many articles, I have tried to practice and demonstrate the philosophy of multidisciplinary interaction. I thank my many friends and coauthors for the opportunity to work with them and for the ideas, willingness, sacrifices, initiative, and patience necessary for the many successes that I have been fortunate to share.

I thank my students at Stonehill College, North Easton, Massachusetts, for the opportunity to learn and share with them. Their questions and concerns have challenged me to gather the knowledge and experiences that have been used to write this book.

Many have helped with the editing of this text. I thank Allan Goldberg, William A. Norko, Jr., Charles Anderson, Susan Cerrone, Lawrence Schmitz, and Warren F. Dahlin, Jr., for their time and insights.

I express a debt of gratitude to my wife, Cathy, and our two sons, Shaun and Timothy, for their understanding of a committed husband and father during the preparation of this book. I thank John Kerrigan for listening during our long distance runs.

Without the help of these people and many others, this book would not have been prepared. For all the errors and omissions, I am indebted to no one but myself.

Finally, I thank long distance running for the health and insights that relieved the aloneness of the long distance runner.

ABOUT THE AUTHOR

Mr. Priest is the central computer resource manager at Brockton Hospital (Brockton, MA). His administrative responsibilities include the computer resource, central patient registration, purchasing, and pharmacy departments. He is an officer in Healthstat, Inc. (Brockton, MA), a software development company. He is a part-time professor at Stonehill College (North Easton, MA) in the department of health-care administration. He was formerly an adjunct professor in the Graduate School of Engineering at Northeastern University (Boston, MA).

Mr. Priest lectures before national organizations. He is the author of over 70 articles dealing with user experiences with health-care computers, and he authored the text *Managing Hospital Information Systems* (Aspen Publications, 1982).

Mr. Priest was formerly employed in the management engineering department of the Rhode Island Hospital (Providence, RI) and the manufacturing division of the General Electric Company (Pittsfield, MA). He received a Master of Science degree in operations research from the University of Rhode Island and a Bachelor of Science degree in industrial engineering from the University of Massachusetts at Amherst.

CHAPTER 1

Introduction and Background

"What is the most useful computer resource in your department?" one might ask the director of medical records. The first response might be the patient case mix information system, which provides answers to almost any question concerning patient mix and demographic characteristics: admitting diagnosis, diagnosis-related group (DRG), length of stay (LOS), age, or sex. This kind of information is used to develop plans concerning the patient population and to predict how well new services will be accepted.

The same question asked of a home health agency manager might elicit the answer, "microcomputer system." This system has graphic and database software to collect and visualize volume and types of services, and it maintains demographic statistics of the patient population. It also helps in documentation and increases office productivity through its word processing capabilities.

A computer operations manager may answer with "the database software for the integrated clinical and financial systems." That, together with the data communications network to each of the nursing stations, is probably used more than any other resource.

These responses are typical; they highlight several points of view that emerge when one tries to define the term "computer resources."

Definition of Computer Resources

Based on the speciality from which it is approached, the term computer resources (CRs) means different things to different people. Asking each manager in an organization to define computer resources will bring as many different answers as there are health-care specialities. Although this does not help when trying to define terms, it is still a real and quite appropriate situation—every specialty has its own objectives. It follows that each specialty will have its own special needs when using computer resources to meet those objectives. The result is that CR services vary widely across an organization in both form and content.

End-users of CRs perceive them primarily as services. End-users see computer resources not so much as the microcomputers and office automation software in their areas, which are viewed as "belonging to the department," but as the central CR staff and the services that they provide. Without always recognizing the fact, end-users are using CRs that include their microcomputers, visual display terminals (VDTs), application software, and printers, as well as the professional CR staff, procedures, and other central CR-provided services.

The user is most keenly aware of the output provided centrally: the operating room schedule, the inventory-on-hand report. The thing that provides the output, or service, has been called the computer system, the information system, and the management information system. Currently, users perceive the central computer area as Computer Resources.

Still others relate CRs to a large database system where all of the organization's shared data are stored and from where they can be retrieved. This idea, while appropriate in principle, has proven unworkable in practice. Several factors work against the single, all-encompassing database approach to providing CR services. Most importantly, the diversification and unique functionality of each specialty's needs make the simplification of all data elements into one database impossible from a practical point of view. Thus, microcomputers offer each specialty a tool to increase productivity and another method to meet its unique needs.

In addition, the financial resources and the sustained, high-level management support required for an all-encompassing, organization-wide computer system are beyond the capabilities of most organizations. Thus, as various users identify the need for computer use, the result is usually multiple computer systems to service those different needs.

To complicate the matter of defining CRs further, a new fact of life in the 1990s must be recognized: While several information systems require CRs to be provided through centralized computer staff, many computer systems are now entirely selected, installed, and managed by a single end-user area.

The end-user's perspective is correct: Microcomputers, VDTs, printers, and the CR staff are the computer resources. The technician's perspective is also correct: Computer hardware, databases, and the central CR staff itself are the computer resources. How can both be correct?

This dilemma is easy to resolve if one considers the chief executive's point of view. For the chief executive officer (CEO), the organization's objectives—not the individual end-user's objectives—are paramount. Computer resources include all computer-related services available to the organization in pursuing its objectives. To the CEO, each end-user's microcomputer is a computer resource, exactly as each end-user perceives. However, CR services do not exist in a vacuum. They are made available either through a central computer resource staff, by the end-user's own staff, or from a source outside the organization such as a vendor or consultant.

Any internal group that provides CR services should itself be considered a computer resource. This means that the telecommunications staff and the office automation staff are also computer resources.

Furthermore, the most important characteristic linking these various groups is the use of computer technology to provide information services. The tools used, such as the computers and the telecommunications channels, must also be considered computer resources. Thus, the technician's point of view is also correct.

The term computer resources has a twofold meaning: first, any computer-related service used by the organization and, second, any hardware, software, and staff used to support those computer services.

Three interesting facts follow from this definition. First, CRs are a means to an end—tools used to meet organizational objectives. All managers, especially senior level managers, must acknowledge this fact.

Second, this definition includes the traditional computer systems, such as accounts receivable, but it is not limited to these; it is open-ended. Also included in the definition are the emerging computer applications such as decision support systems (e.g., financial modeling), office automation (e.g., teleconferences), and information center (microcomputer training and application support).

Finally, it should be clear that a computer resource can be either manual or automated. As a practical matter, however, the term computer resources implies the use of the computer.

Users of Computer Resources

The User

The terms "end-user" and "user" are interchangeable in identifying the ultimate user of the CR service. End-users represent a diverse cross section: secretaries, technicians, clerks, physicians, department heads, senior management, and the CEO.

The Used

The output from the CR is information. It is interesting to consider just what it is that end-users actually use.

It was previously suggested that the director of medical records used information to help answer questions about patient preference or to help make decisions about which services to offer. Likewise, the home health agency manager in the example used information from the microcomputer to help document and identify areas in which to focus efforts and to help maintain agency statistics. Clearly, what is being used is information, or the output from the individual CR. However, there are other kinds of computer resources.

For instance, consider the for-profit multihospital chain, which may use the organization's teleconference facilities to exchange information and solve problems with others who are hundreds of miles away. A purchasing agent may reorder inventory by having a microcomputer "talk" with a vendor's large scale computer. In these two cases, the teleconference facilities and the telecommunications network are used to exchange information.

In the first two cases, it was the information produced that was ultimately important, but in the latter cases the resources themselves played the prominent role. Once again, computer resources can be thought of as either the service to the user (i.e., the information produced) or the supportive hardware, software, and staff (i.e., telecommunications and a microcomputer network).

Interaction

Not all computer resources have been successful. Many have failed to achieve the advantages that a computerized information system should offer. It has become clear in studying the disappointments and the success stories of computer resources that the single most critical factor for success is the effective involvement and interaction of the end-users and the computer resource specialists.

Formerly, systems problems were blamed on the computer. "The computer made a mistake" was a common response. Today it is recognized that it is people who make the mistakes. The user may have instructed the system incorrectly, a technician might have entered data incorrectly, the nurse supervisor might not have clearly explained what was needed, or the laboratory technologist might have verified incomplete or inaccurate results. This is a new world for many users, and it can be a bewildering one because of the complexity and jargon that may accompany a computer resource.

End-users need to understand the principles of computer resources and their own essential role in computer system development and use. In the same sense, the central CR staff must practice the role of a support function and not dictate the use and restriction of CR systems and services to the users. Both the users and the central CR staff must understand their roles in the development, use, and evolution of computer resources. They must attempt to do this without fear of the jargon that adds to the complexity of computer systems; it is critical that all CR users appreciate this basic premise. To maintain and use CRs continuously and successfully, both the end-user and the CR staff must be held jointly accountable for the computer resources.

Many users have fears about the introduction of a computer system in their environment. The best way to overcome these fears is to understand the concepts underlying computer systems and to gain experience in the definition, design, installation, and control of computer systems (Priest, 1986). The person most responsible for developing and controlling the system must understand the various techniques to remove any communications gap between the CR professionals and the end-user. People involved with the computer must understand the responsibilities of using computer resources and the various approaches to CR planning and management. The users should especially focus on those areas of CR that they manage, independent of the central CR staff.

Today, computer resource opportunities extend beyond the scope of the central CR manager's control. This is cause for both the central CR staff and the users to examine each other's role and responsibilities in the growth and use of CR. Technological advances in hardware and software are having a direct impact on all operating areas, often resulting in changes in the quality of patient services and in the cost of organizational service. For example, where real-time processing was once only for organizations with large budgets, today's technology "painlessly" offers that service to physicians' offices, nursing homes, home care agencies, and virtually any size organization. Real-time and batch services, in-house staff services, and outside vendor microcomputer and mainframe services are now making the CR cost-justifiable, if not mandatory, for all.

Answers to specific questions about the right mix of in-house and outside services, end-user control of CRs, acquisition of microcomputers, etc., require knowledge of an organization's size, structure, location, resources, history, politics, and other factors. A primary requirement for the successful application of CRs to meet end-users' needs is the understanding of people interaction. This idea of interaction will be expanded upon in Chapter 3.

The Development of Computer Resouces

The Stages of Computer Resources

Historical discussions are often not emphasized in business computer texts. The reader is given a brief introduction to Babbage, von Neumann, and others responsible for the early development of computers (Sullivan

1988, 491–508). Furthermore, if one is aware of these people and of the key advances in technology such as transistors, integrated circuitry, large scale integration, very large scale integration, and parallel processing, one often assumes that a focus on the current environment is the only productive focus. However, these assumptions overlook some important lessons.

A glimpse at the development of the computer as a user resource, from the user's point of view, can provide substantial rewards. Even in the environment of the late 1980s, it is not difficult to find examples of organizations that exist in different periods of CR development. Recognizing where an organization lies along the historical path of CR development can assist one in taking full advantage of CR capabilities and in planning how to change for the future.

A small nursing home, for example, may still rely on batch processing and focus on automating only data processing applications such as payroll and patient billing. A hospital may be in the early phases of the development of real-time CR capability. Hospital personnel may be developing a patient computer system to maintain and retrieve records of past patient visits (i.e., allergies, next of kin, previous dates of service or treatment, physician, etc.), radiology transcripts, laboratory and pharmacy profiles for the current service visit, and historical records of case mix to aid planning and scheduling of future services.

A physician's office may rely on the use of microcomputers for billing and maintaining a patient profile and visit file. The physician may also have access to a hospital's large mainframe computer with telecommunication and database software (allowing the microcomputers to access large files) to download patient data from the hospital to the office microcomputers periodically. A large-organization chain may have implemented a distributed data-processing architecture. Each chief financial officer (CFO) might have a microcomputer that is in almost constant contact with the home office computer, transferring information about both the current financial status and projected areas of concern and investigation. The home office, in addition to various other CR services, might provide an information center to meet ad hoc end-user information needs.

Clearly, organizations today exist in various stages of CR development. Each of these stages seems to provide different capabilities to end-users, and each seems to be able to be implemented using different organizational strategies.

The increased sophistication of end-users, the increased demand for more and more immediate access to management information, and recent technological advances have brought about an entirely new paradigm of CR use in organizations. Information is now not only a means to an end, a tool for managers to use in meeting their objectives; it is now considered a resource to be managed. Making information available and maintaining it has become an end in itself. The way to manage this resource is to manage the channels for capturing, maintaining, and making information accessible.

In the 1980s, several different hardware and software developments have begun to converge, seemingly with one, formerly unobtainable objective: to make needed information immediately available to managers, wherever they may be located and whenever they may need it. Microcomputers have given end-users significant control over their immediate, internal, information-processing environment. Information centers and fourth generation programming languages allow end-users to modify their microcomputer output dynamically as their management needs change. Downloading from host computers onto user-controlled microcomputers has been especially useful in making broadly available such quantitative techniques as modeling. Telecommunications capabilities and distributed data processing (DP) architectures now allow the users' computer resources to grow and change as the physical structure of the organization grows and changes. Optical disks using lasers to store and retrieve large amounts of data make possible a paperless medical record of present and past patient medical history which is available immediately to all specialties.

In the 1980s, the direction has not shifted from the basic concept of the management information system. That is, the direction has not shifted away from the idea of providing past, current, and future windows of information. Instead, there has been an expansion of this very successful idea. Instead of making these windows of information available for different sectors of the organization individually, the aim is to make them available across the entire organization, bounded neither by the frustrating time lag of the central computer department nor by the physical remoteness of some of the components of the organization.

In addition to the traditionally defined information systems, the 1980s have witnessed the emergence of an entirely new class of CR services. Office automation, including word processing, teleconferencing, electronic mail, automated records management, and other services, has been strongly influenced by the behaviorists. Not considering the marketing bonanza for the vendors of office automation equipment, we can see that users have adopted these new services for good reason. The goal is to make the office worker more productive and to motivate white-collar workers by providing the latest and best tools for the job. This directly reflects the principles of behaviorism.

Health-care organizations are currently in the beginning stages of this latest change, as can be seen by the view of information and its use held by organizations. Consequently, at times it seems that there are more questions than there are answers. For example, how will the traditional information systems be managed now that virtually any end-user has the capability (through the use of microcomputers) of constructing its own systems? How and by whom are the emerging computer resources to be managed?

These questions are difficult to answer. There is no one solution that is right for every organization. Once aware of the problems, one must consider the open-ended strategies that enhance the search for solutions to these problems in the individual organization. The questions are difficult to answer, but they cannot be avoided.

The Value of Data

Data are a vital ingredient to good management. The fact that data are now associated with computers has a part in the history and growth of CRs. Senior and line management certainly recognize data as essential resources of the organization. Being essential resources, data have value and worth; determining this worth can be a complex task. However, there are two things about data of which you can be sure: the quantity of data and the demand for data are both increasing. These increases force one to place values and priorities on data based on economic and technological constraints; there are limits to data storage and the allowable cost of storing and retrieving data.

Data have both cost-associated values and time-associated values. The cost values can be seen when one considers two sources of data coming into an office. One tells that John Smith has worked two hours overtime; the other says that if a valve is not adjusted, a patient's life will be in jeopardy. Which piece of data has the largest worth and priority? How much should be invested in hardware, software, and labor to make data available?

Data also have a time value. If information is requested, is the answer required immediately or is it permissible to wait to retrieve the data? What timeframe is allowed for retrieval—instantly or within a certain range of time? Based on cost of storage and retrieval, what data should be available immediately, and what should be available later?

Before computers, data needs were kept very simple because of the complexities and timeliness of retrieving and analyzing data. Today, automation provides access to effective utilization of data, and the cost, timeliness, and priority of data have become factors in the determination and usage of computer resources.

Summary

If one considers the history of computer resource management from the point of view of the end-user, new insights might be gained. The use of computer resources has progressed meaningfully in organizations. According to the DP view, computers are used primarily to give management an accurate view of the current state of the organization. DP just processes data—it does nothing with the results. According to the management information system (MIS) view, computers provide three windows of information—past, current, and future. The MIS informs management. Finally, the CR view encourages expansion of the MIS view, making information immediately accessible without regard for geographic boundaries.

It is possible to progress to a mature CR paradigm when one accepts that communications and shared responsibilities between the end-users and the central computer group are essential. It also seems that the change in management's focus from output to people has spurred many of the most recent technological developments. Finally, the emergence of the microcomputer, optical disks, and the availability of universal telecommunication capabilities and other such recent advances in technology have assisted in the emergence of an entirely new set of computer resource services. Clearly, many factors have contributed to the development of the use of computers in organizations.

None of the stages of computer resource development has disappeared from society. It is still easy to find different organizations that exist, whether appropriately or not, in any of the stages of CR development. If an organization is just beginning its encounter with computer resources, it can, if it wishes, follow along the historical path. An organization can begin by implementing DP applications, expand to develop MIS capabilities, and in the future move toward the CR view.

Organizations need not be forced to relive this history however. With currently available technology, it is entirely possible, with appropriate foresight and planning, for an organization to begin with the CR perspective. In fact, this is recommended. It is the CR perspective that takes into account all of the lessons learned by the prior two generations of end-users.

Finally, as has been mentioned, there are still many unanswered questions. Where, for example, should an organization with geographically dispersed components place the management and location of computer resources? It seems clear that there will be no universal answers. Users will do well to understand the questions and work out answers that are at least consistent with past experiences.

Computer Resources Within the Organizational Structure

History

In the late 1950s and the early 1960s, computer resources were located mostly in large hospitals and other large health-care facilities in the form of mainframe computer hardware and software. Staff resided essentially in two primary areas: the data processing department, which served the financial department's processing needs with batch processing, and the laboratory, with its minicomputers processing patient tests. Each end-user area maintained sole control over its computer resources. Computer usage was confined to those users with budgets and prominence. In addition, the major software available addressed only financial and laboratory applications.

In the mid-1960s, two developments caused a policy of strict adherence to the centralization of computer resources. First, the larger computers that the manufacturers were selling presented economies of scale that organizations with limited budgets could not ignore. Computers and professional staff were so expensive that organizations mandated the central location of these services. This meant that no end-user could acquire or manage its own computer resources.

Second, organizations realized that proven software applications were limited and, in determining where to spend money and development resources, the information needs of the financial users were given first priority. A centralized DP section would allow senior management to both monitor information needs and control organization-wide use of CRs to meet these needs.

Until the late 1970s, the central DP or MIS section was the main location for computer resources. Microcomputers were located primarily in the financial user areas. Some word processors, the predecessors of microcomputers with another name, were not yet recognized organization-wide as computer resources. Also, DP or MIS personnel almost always reported to the chief financial officer of the organization, historically the first end-user and one who maintained strong control of the so-called existing computer resources.

Today, professionals in administration, home care, physician office practice, nursing, public relations, finance, human resources, and various other support and ancillary areas require an understanding of the capabilities of computer resources. Users are sophisticated and at ease with computers, and demand for computer resources is expected from all end-users. In the late 1980s, technology supplied cost-effective solutions that call for decentralization of these resources. However, the need for organization-wide maintenance, planning, and support of these services has kept the centralized concept of the CR staff, but forced its accessibility beyond the financial user area.

A Partner Equal in Importance to Its Users

How should today's computer resources fit into the organizational structure? Where is the central CR responsibility in the organizational chart? These are really two separate questions. First, where should the computer resources physically reside in the organization and, second, what are the lines of responsibility?

The answer to the second question has been provided in prior sections of this chapter. It is critical that senior management recognize that the path to successful usage of CRs lies along the road of cooperation and joint accountability between the central CR support area and the end-user areas. The central CR function serves the total organization and, to succeed, must be a partner equal in importance to each of those with whom it must assume this joint accountability. Central CR staff should be accountable as members of the senior management team.

This view is also consistent with historical developments. Although advances in technology have in many cases eliminated the economies of scale of the large computers, there is a need for central computer hardware and software resources. Technological advances have provided senior management with a need for real-time access to organization information. A central CR staff meets those needs.

User-managed Resources

The answer to the question of user accountability follows a different line of logic. End-user areas are educated depending on their needs for CRs and therefore must be as responsible as the central CR staff in the development of CRs for their own use. Where should the resources reside? With the users.

Cautions

Valid arguments against user control of the physical resources quickly emerge. Some users may not be educated relative to their responsibilities in this management role. Some may not have the technical staff or knowledge; some may not have the desire to assume these additional responsibilities. The users might not want to or be capable of managing these resources.

Further, if users do assume this function, the infamous Frankenstein monster of uncontrolled modification and change is loose. Once the resources (hardware, software, staff) reside with the user, how can changes to those resources be controlled?

Also, there are CR systems and services that are multiuser by nature and should not be controlled by only one of the users because that one user is likely to take too narrow a view of the use of that system or service (e.g., shared multiuser databases, information centers).

Indeed, there are many who would argue that user management of computer resources will almost never work and should always be approached with caution. Although this path should always be approached with caution, it should be cautiously implemented, not cautiously deterred.

The Principle

These objections cannot be ignored. Many well-meaning plans for allowing users more control of computer resources have ended in disaster for these very reasons. These problems, however, are problems in implementation, not in principle. The general principle is that the computer resources should be managed as close to the users as possible, and the direction of that management task should be a goal of the central CR staff. There must be central planning and direction and also maximal individual user authority.

The idea of additional control over one's objectives is a strong motivating influence for users to want to manage their own computer resources. Often users are quite willing to acquire additional education and gain some experiential knowledge of CRs in order to manage their own CRs. However, the central CR staff must play the more demanding role of planning, implementing, and also managing the ongoing use and maintenance of the CR system. The central CR staff must assist the users in their task, if necessary, and also be prepared to recognize those users not attending to organization objectives, policies, and direction. This certainly should be the exception, not the rule.

The role of overseeing the use of the output of the system and of planning for the future use of the system still falls to the User Computer Resource Manager (UCRM). The user area must play a prominent role in the use of CRs, even if that role does not include bringing those resources physically into the area. Any potential user who does not recognize this need for interaction should be avoided. To do otherwise would be to court disaster.

The Central CR Role

What, then, is the main role of the central CR staff? Planning and services! The central group establishes the framework in which these satellite areas exist. The central CR staff is responsible for identifying and promoting the global view of the computer needs of the organization. Once these needs are identified, the central CR staff must recognize changes, bring them to the attention of senior and user management, and assist in their implementation and usage.

A central CR manager who sits as a partner with end-users provides each end-user with equal opportunity to utilize limited CR budgets and staff as judged by what is best for the organization, not for an individual end-user. This senior position also provides the opportunity for organization-wide access to clinical, administrative, and financial applications and data. Figure 1-1 is one example of how the central CR manager serves as a member of senior management within the organizational structure and of the many services that the CR staff provides to end-users. The central CR staff can serve the special needs of each area while managing a common database for the information needs of senior and middle management. These issues will be discussed in greater depth in Chapters 7 and 8.

The Solution

The organizational structure, then, has computer resources residing in the user areas whenever appropriate. In addition, the role of all CR managers is to search out and help develop these appropriate situations.

Further, the central CR staff has a twofold role. First, it provides senior management with an organizational mechanism for the monitoring of needs and the planning and selecting of resource use. Second, the central CR area, appropriately, has many of the computer resources physically located within its confines to assist users in meeting their individual specialty information needs using shared resources.

To maximize the central CR staff's effectiveness within the organization, management must present the function as a partner equal to all user areas. This means positioning the CR manager at an organizational level equal to that of the managers of areas served by computer resources.

On the other side of the token, the physical location of the actual resources need not be central. The users should manage the CRs whenever possible. Although this approach has certain inherent risks, it should nonetheless be cautiously implemented. It is possible to link strong central control and direction with individual user autonomy.

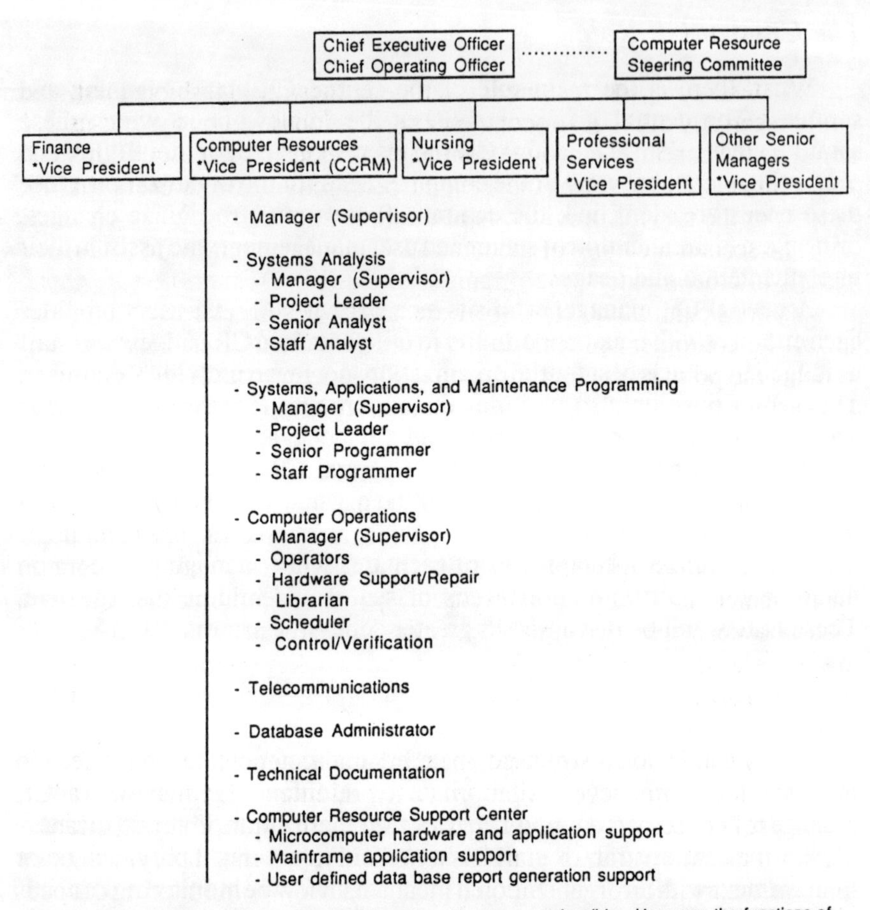

Figure 1-1. The central computer resource manager (CCRM) as a member of senior management and the various central CR staff positions which provide end-user services.

Conclusion

The term computer resources is defined in a twofold fashion. First, CRs could mean any of the microcomputer applications used by the end-user. It could be the centrally managed computer accessed by the user with VDTs and printers. This reflects the general perspective of end-users that the output, or the service provided is of ultimate importance.

The second meaning of the term CR includes all hardware (minicomputers, microcomputers, mainframe computers, VDTs, printers, telecommunications equipment, etc.), software, and professional staff that provide all of the computer systems and services to the end-user. This meaning reflects the point of view of the central CR function that is responsible for the management of the use of these resources in pursuit of the organization's strategic business plan and objectives.

In the current CR environment, end-users use not only the information output from central computers, but also many of the computer resource facilities provided through microcomputers managed solely by end-users. One of the primary principles that users and CR professionals must observe in implementing CRs successfully is the principle of interaction. Cooperation between these two groups, support for each other's objectives and needs (related to CRs), and the acceptance of a policy of joint accountability for CR success or failure are attitudes and experiences that must be demanded and promoted.

Early computer use focused on speed and accuracy; the computer was seen as a tool to massage available data to present management with an up-to-date reflection of the current state of the organization. Later applications drew on a combination of management theory, systems theory, and information theory. New uses emerged. The MIS view held that the computer should not be limited to providing managers with an understanding of the current state of the organization, but should also be able to recall past experiences and use past and current data to try to forecast the future.

The CR view expands upon the MIS view. In addition to providing the three windows of information (past, present, and future), computers and other support technology (now as a group called computer resources) should make information immediately accessible to managers wherever they may be and whenever they may want to use it.

Data have both cost-associated and time-associated values and must be managed as a corporate asset. The computer resources function must be recognized in the organization as a partner to the areas that are served. The manager of the CR staff must be a senior management team member who is involved in the organization's long-range planning and who directs computer resources toward the organization's strategic goals. Chapter 2 discusses the people most responsible for managing computer resources.

Questions and Assignment

Questions

1. The local community hospital uses the Bell Telemarketing System, advertised on TV, to increase patient awareness of preventive medicine methods such as breast exams and annual physicals. Explain why this is or is not a computer resource.
2. The local visiting nurses association is entering the computer age. The agency administrator feels secure that automation of the payroll and billing functions will be successful. Until these applications have been fully implemented, however, he is refusing to consider other possible applications. Given the discussion in the text of the historical path that users of information systems have followed, explain why this is or is not a good management strategy.

Assignment

Break into small groups of two to five students each. Each team should identify a local health-care provider or other organization for research. A department or division of a large organization will work just as well. Each group should make contact with and research the target organization relative to the following questions: What are the current computer resources? Where is this organization in its historical development in the use of CRs? What position does the CR function hold in the structure of the organization?

After this research is completed, each team should identify recommendations for change and present a report to the class.

Suggested Readings

Arnold, W.V. 3rd, and M.A. Leonard. Spring 1987. HMOs and PPOs: an operational guide. Topics *in Healthcare Finance* 13(3): 19–31.

Austin, C.J. 1988. *Information systems for health services administration.* Ann Arbor, MI: Health Administration Press.

Catchpole, P., D. Avison, and S. Peart. August 26–September 1, 1987. Computers in nursing news. The tale of two systems. *Nursing Times* 83(34): 57–58.

Coleman, J.R., and C.E. Lowry. June 1983. A computerized MIS to support the administration of quality patient care in HMOs organized as IPAs. *Journal of Medical Systems* 7(3): 273–284.

Drazen, E.L., and N.L. Moorse. March 1986. Use of computerized information systems in U.S. health maintenance organizations and hospitals. *Computer Methods and Programs in Biomedicine* 22(1): 105–110.

Grams, R.R., G.C. Peck, J.R. Massey, et al. August 1985. Review of hospital data processing in the United States (1982–1984). *Journal of Medical Systems* 175–269.

Harrison, M., and B. Green. April 1986. The computer in health visiting. *Midwife Health Visit and Community Nurse* 22(4): 110–114.

Kapp, M.B. March 1986. Preventing malpractice suits in long term care facilities. *Quality Review Bulletin* 12(3): 109–113.

Kennedy, O.G. March 20, 1988. Multis seek alternative care system automation. *Hospitals* 62(6): 104.

Kenny, J.C. March–April 1988. The use of computers in community health. *Nurse Education* 13(2): 22.

Martin, K. October 1987. A client classification system adaptable for computerization. *National League of Nursing Publication* 191–196.

Muller, J.H. November 1986. MIS software brings hi–tech care home. *Nursing Management* 17(11): 48–50.

Muller, J.H. March–April 1987. Medical information systems for home care. *Home Healthcare Nursing* 5(2): 23–27.

Packer, C.L. July 20, 1987. Information systems lack flexibility: HMOs. *Hospitals* 61(4): 82.

Peters, T.J., and R.H. Waterman, Jr. 1982. *In search of excellence*. New York: Harper and Row.

Priest, S.L. October 1986. Understanding your organization's computer resources. *The Healthcare Supervisor* 5(1): 24–40.

Prussin, J.A. December 1987. Automation: the competitive edge for HMOs and other alternative delivery systems. *Journal of Medical Systems* 11(6): 431–444.

Rantz, M.J. April 1988. Resources for long–term care. *Journal of Gerontology Nursing* 14(4): 35–39.

Roundtable on information management. June 1988. Information management: emergence of a new deal. *Journal of the Healthcare Financial Management Association.*

Saba, V.K., and K.A. McCormick. 1986. *Essentials of computers for nurses.* Philadelphia: Lippincott.

Schank, M.J., L.D. Doney, and S.C. Ross. May–June 1986. Use of a data base system by a home health care agency: an illustrative example. *Home Healthcare Nursing* 4(3): 22–28.

Stein, K.Z., and D.G. Eigsti. April 1987. Evaluating the use of a data base system for community health nursing students. *Journal of Nursing Education* 26(4): 162–163.

Sullivan, D.R., T.G. Lewis, and C.R. Cook. 1988. *Computing today: microcomputer concepts and applications.* 2d ed. 491–508. Boston: Houghton Mifflin Co.

Wright, C. September 1985. Computer–aided nursing diagnosis for community health nurses. *Nursing Clinics of North America* 20(3): 487–495.

CHAPTER 2

The Computer Resource Managers

Introduction

Who in the organization should be responsible for managing the computer resources? In principle, the answer could be threefold: it is each of the user computer resource managers (UCRMs); it is the central computer resource manager (CCRM); it is both the UCRMs and the CCRM. The depth of relationships among the UCRMs and the CCRM determines the scope and utilization of computer resources in an organization. The path to successful computer resources lies along the road of cooperation, joint responsibility, and individual accountability.

Structurally, this interactive relationship might be described by a network with many modes (Figure 2-1). Interacting with all nodes is the node of the Central Computer Resource Manager (CCRM). The other nodes are the individual User Computer Resource Managers (UCRMs). The relationship that binds the node of the CCRM and the individual nodes of each UCRM is twofold. First are the computers and services that are available to the users. Just as important, however, are the communication and joint responsibility and accountability of the CCRM and the various UCRMs. Clearly, each node can stand alone but, with separate nodes, the network is weak. The strength of the network is the ability of each node to respect the other and its contribution to the total organization.

Who are these people? What should their backgrounds be? What are their management profiles? With the answers to these questions, the reader will understand more completely the role of computer resource (CR) managers. Just as important, these answers will serve as guidelines for the selection of future CR managers.

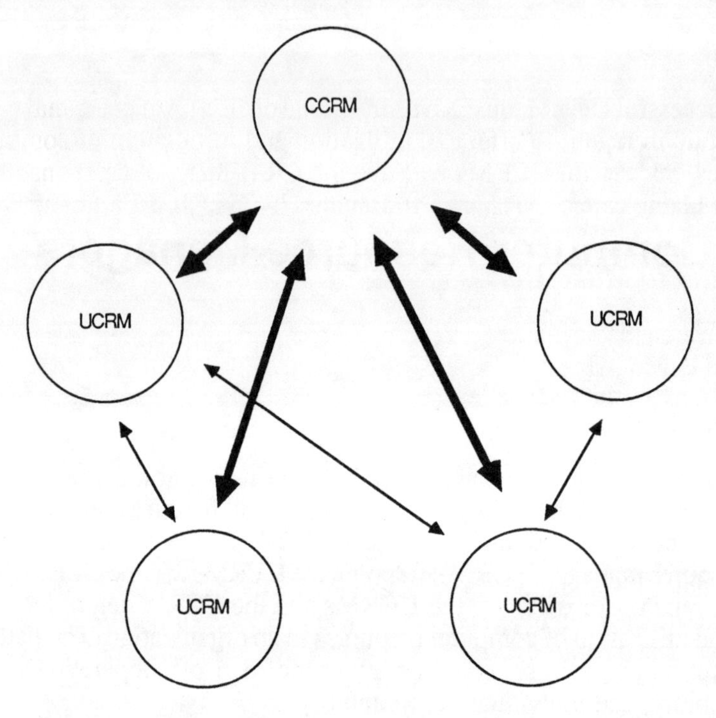

The fine two-way arrows indicate regular dialogue between user computer resource managers (UCRM) who share data and applications. The bold two-way arrows indicate a central computer resource manager (CCRM) maintaining dialogue with all UCRMs. The absense of a line between two UCRMs recognizes that some users may not have a need to routinely communicate with one another.

Figure 2-1. Interactive relationships among central and user computer resource managers.

The User Computer Resource Manager (UCRM)

A Member of the User Staff

An organization has many user computer resource managers. Each end-user area will have a UCRM. This person most generally will combine the computer responsibility with other responsibilities. The UCRM could be a supervisor, a senior member of the user staff, or the user area manager.

Attitude

A successful UCRM must have an attitude of "it's up to me to make this successful" in regard to effective utilization and installation of computer resources. Successful UCRMs feel that the CR is their sole responsibility and that blame cannot be shared or assumed by the CR department.

Authority to Make Decisions

In an area that is introducing computer resources to its staff for the first time and in which these resources will play a major role in helping to meet user objectives, the UCRM responsibilities will initially be assumed by the user manager. The UCRM must have the authority to make decisions and changes. This authority can later be delegated to another senior staff member of the area, but initial automation forces many user area changes and causes a redefinition of how needs are to be met. Decisions must be made quickly and with knowledge of their consequences. These responsibilities must be assumed by a person with the authority to make the technical, process, and management decisions that will arise. Experience has shown that the introduction of major computer changes in an area works best with end-user senior management guiding the process.

CRs and services are successful when the UCRM takes an active and aggressive role in the use and management of the CRs. The UCRM must develop and maintain a user environment that allows this to happen.

Maintain Communications among Users

The UCRM must ensure communication among all members of the user area as well as interact with other UCRMs who share mutual CRs. For example, the laboratory UCRM must let the laboratory staff know what application changes are being addressed, must listen to their concerns and fears, and must be a champion for their ideas and problems. In addition, the UCRM will be in contact with the nursing UCRM and will discuss mutual concerns, such as cancelled and duplicate laboratory orders and the prompt reporting of laboratory results.

The UCRM must be able to identify changes and problems in the user CRs and to prescribe solutions. The UCRM must listen to the staff that is using the CRs. The UCRM must communicate changes and problems to the central CR manager and use the available centralized CRs as needed.

Computer Literacy

One is best prepared to assume CR responsibilities if one is computer-literate. This does not mean having to be a microcomputer expert, but it does mean having an understanding of the terms frequently associated with computer resources, such as hardware, software, real-time, etc. A person can be prepared by both experience and conceptual understanding. A UCRM should have a sound, basic understanding of computers and information resources, along with a grasp of prior successes and failures of computer resources in similar user areas and organizations.

The successful UCRM will have an understanding of the capabilities and limits of computer resources. He or she must know how the end-user currently operates and its specific needs and procedures, and must participate actively in CR usage.

Documentation

UCRMs must document the progress, successes, and failures of the CRs. They must ensure that user manuals are prepared. They can ensure good communication among users by documenting problems and processes so that all can understand or disagree. The written word is a commitment and a definition. It ensures that all areas of responsibility are covered, or indeed lets others see that areas are not covered. It assigns responsibility. Essentially, documentation communicates to all with a need to know.

A UCRM can conduct a detailed analysis and documentation of user needs, contribute to both the hardware and software selection decisions, test new resources and services, prepare user methods and procedures, and train users. To be able to perform these tasks, the UCRM must intimately understand the needs and responsibilities of the area.

Utilization of Central Computer Resources

A UCRM will effectively use the central computer resources. For example, microcomputer assistance and training may be provided by the central information center. The central CR staff can support the UCRM by providing technical expertise to investigate central computer response problems and ensuring proper preventive and remedial maintenance on microcomputers, VDTs and printers. Other services provided centrally would be additional hardware capability, such as computer access lines and telecommunication links with outside services.

A UCRM will often use the CR staff as a sounding board for ideas and process concerns. System analysis professionals can lend insight and provide alternative solutions for system concerns and problems.

In summary, the user computer resources manager should:

- Be a member of the user area
- Be computer-literate
- Understand the process of the user area
- Feel that "It's up to me to make this successful"
- Have the authority to make decisions
- Maintain communications among users
- Be a documentation type person
- Effectively use central CRS

The Central Computer Resource Manager (CCRM)

Background

A central computer resource manager is part of the organization's senior management team. The role of a CCRM is to provide guidance and recommendations for the allocation and use of the organization's computer resources. The CCRM should understand the health-care business and be knowledgeable about the design and application of computer technology. The CCRM will assist the UCRM to improve productivity and to keep the cost of computer resources down while purchasing all of the computer resources necessary to meet the needs of the organization's strategic business plan (Packer 1988).

The CCRM should have a blend of management, application, and technical skills developed through academic and experiential learning. The CCRM will have administrative responsibility for the central CR staff and will also be responsible for coordinating the growth and use of computer resources throughout the organization. This latter responsibility requires the CCRM to have a genuine sensitivity to user needs and also be capable of promoting the larger corporate perspective. The CCRM must develop and maintain an environment that fosters interaction with the users (Rydell 1988).

Computer resources cannot be viewed solely from the departmental perspective. The impact of an end-user's computer resources on the organization must be understood and recognized. For example, a hospital might use a minicomputer for clinical and financial applications. In addition, the utilization review (UR) area might use a microcomputer database application. This approach meets both organization-wide needs and UR needs. If the UR microcomputer needs to access minicomputer data, however, problems could arise if the micro is not capable of "talking" to the minicomputer. These problems would be avoided if the CCRM has established a policy that requires that microcomputers be compatible with central services. Often, personnel, equipment, and interuser problems can be anticipated from the CCRM's view of the organization.

To carry this example further, the CCRM may also perceive that the data utilized by the UR department will soon be required for governmental analysis. Thus, the departmental perspective needs to be seen, but the global view of the CCRM is necessary for planning and setting organizational goals.

Computer Resource Culture

The CCRM is the person primarily responsible for developing and maintaining the computer resource "culture." That is, this person is responsible for identifying CR objectives and accomplishing them, for establishing attitudes about successes and failures, and for developing frameworks for initiating and undertaking projects. In short, the CCRM is responsible for establishing an environment that allows and encourages the necessary interactive relationship with the end-users.

The CCRM must have a genuine sensitivity to end-user operations and concerns. Successful organizations realize that the CR staff can best respond to user needs only through a real understanding of the users and their responsibilities. Conversely, users who are aware of the CR commitment to successful computer resources do not hesitate to initiate discussions of systems problems. This team approach is a necessary condition precedent to successful systems (Rockart 1982).

The CR staff serves the organization through effective dialogue with user areas. A demonstrated interest in understanding user needs and problems prevents barriers to communications and "finger pointing." User managers and CR managers must communicate in system selection, design, and implementation.

Internal Communication

It is critical that the CCRM maintain a continual dialogue with the staff of the CR area, both to understand their concerns and to share and learn from their experiences and insights. For this to happen, staff must be informed (as much as possible) of user area and organizational plans. This quells rumors and opens two-way communication that results in more dedicated subordinates and a more informed CCRM.

This internal communication can be further enhanced through staff meetings and by routing pertinent literature and reports through the staff. Staff must feel that they are part of the organization; they should participate in meetings particular to their interest and feel free to make suggestions and recommendations to the CCRM.

Technical Skills

The technical skills of the CCRM are not of foremost importance. Experience has shown that problems arise when a CCRM is more concerned with keeping up with state-of-the-art hardware and software than with understanding departmental changes and organizational needs.

Technical knowledge is important. Although it enables the CCRM to communicate with those CR personnel who are technically oriented, it could hinder communications with the senior and middle management teams. This dichotomy of views between senior management and a technically oriented CCRM most frequently arises when the CCRM has a strong programming and computer operations orientation and little systems and administrative background.

Communication Skills

The CCRM must display effective oral, written, and presentation communications skills. This individual will be responsible for making clear the direction and intent of computer resources management for the organization. The successful executive in this role must have marketing and public relations skills and be able to provide senior management, users, and the entire organizational community with an awareness and understanding of CR capabilities, direction, and performance.

Senior management is output-oriented. The CCRM must therefore be able to make effective presentations to senior management. These presentations should clarify the availability and use of computer resources and describe how these systems and services address the organization's strategic business plan.

A CCRM must have an academic understanding of and experiential use of management, organization, systems, and information theory and must also have oral presentation and writing skills to strengthen the components of his/her professional portfolio. These principles and skills are discussed in courses in business administration, but they must be developed and honed through use in the organization.

The Business Plan

The computer resource plan must be linked to the organization's business plan. Computer resources must be able to perform in response to expanding needs. The CCRM must therefore be allowed to comment on the organization's business plan and be part of its development. Computer resources are critical to the success of today's organization, and the CCRM should be involved in strategic business planning in order to carry out the expanding and critical role of CRs.

The CCRM must prepare an annual report on how the organization's CRs are meeting the organization's strategic business plan. This report will include the status of the year's CR projects and the cost of providing CR services.

Project Orientation

Because of the relatively large amount of money and hours that could be expended in constructing and implementing even a simple computer system, most of these undertakings are managed as projects. The CR undertakings are managed as a group of interrelated tasks, each with assigned, estimated, targeted completion dates and costs. The CCRM should have demonstrated project management experience.

This experiential background is necessary because the leading cause of project cost and time overruns is project management. It is difficult to produce estimates for systems development projects. Application development and implementation tasks should be well defined. In addition, there are often many interrelationships in CR project that require a diversity of experience and user sensitivity.

In addition to managing projects, the CCRM is responsible for planning the breadth and scope of projects that the organization will undertake. This means negotiating the CR budget in line with the organization's strategic business plan. This adds a further burden. The CCRM must establish standards for project initiation, project scheduling, and project evaluation to best utilize the limited staff and financial resources available.

In summary, the central computer resources manager should:

- Be a member of the senior management team
- Maintain, promote, and purchase CRs in line with the organizational strategic business plan
- Be sensitive to user needs

- Have a balanced background
  - — Technical skills
  - — Project orientation
  - — Presentation and communication skills
- Perform an annual CR performance assessment
- Develop an annual CR long-range and short-range plan after reviewing the organizational strategic business plan

The Steering Committee

A computer resources steering committee is necessary in an organization that will select, implement, and maintain computer resources. In any organization, there is competition for limited CR budgets and staff, and the committee will have the important task of determining major computer project priorities. Further, it will be responsible for requiring and encouraging participatory interaction between the end-users and the central CR staff.

Members

The steering committee is composed of senior and line management representatives who have visibility at all levels of the organization. Because the computer resources services being considered will have an impact on the achievement of organizational objectives, CR projects must be carefully defined and given priority relative to their impact on the organization's strategic plan.

A steering committee will generally include six to eight people such as the Chief Executive Officer (CEO), the Chief Operating Officer (COO), and Vice Presidents of finance, nursing, computer resources, medical staff, and trustees. Although the committee will not be directly responsible for providing funding for the acquisition of computer resources, its membership must include individuals who are able to represent computer resource funding when appropriate. For example, trustees who also serve on the finance committee and planning committee will be able to put into perspective the role of computer resources in the funding and planning priority process. As a group, these people should reflect the personality and the goals of the organization.

In some organizations, it may appear that the CEO, and even the COO, are too busy with other areas of concern to be able to be committee members. A word of caution here: in today's expanding environment, the impact of computer resources is organization-wide, and CRs are essential in meeting an organization's strategic business plan, for which the CEO and COO are held accountable. Thus, if it is determined that one or both of these two key individuals cannot make time available, there must be other methods, such as routine updates on committee meetings and agendas, to include these individuals. A decision not to include the CEO or COO must not be made hastily.

Depending on the size of the organization, the CEO may be the chairperson of the committee, but another senior executive, such as the COO, may chair the group. Other organizations may appoint the Chief Financial Officer or even the CCRM as chairperson. Having the CCRM chair the committee may not be preferred because this may give the impression that the committee is serving only the more narrow role of a CR sounding board.

Frequently, senior management has time pressures and competing priorities that make it less effective in guiding computer resource decisions. Getting senior management participation in the meetings can be a challenge for the CCRM. It is important to plan the meetings appropriately to maximize usage of senior management time. This preparation includes individual meetings with committee members before steering committee meetings to ensure that their concerns are properly addressed and understood before the meetings. All meetings should have a specific agenda. The agenda, prior meeting minutes, and other back-up information should be distributed before the meeting.

The frequency of the meetings can be an important factor in senior management participation. The timing of the meeting must address needed issues and not simply satisfy a meeting schedule. The steering committee of an organization deciding on a major computer conversion may meet more frequently than that of one with an established computer system.

The CCRM should maintain the minutes of the meetings. This allows the CCRM to be more in contact with members and to coordinate the agenda of the meetings. The CCRM should be required regularly to update the committee on the state of computer resources in the organization.

Other ad hoc representatives may be called upon as the committee deems necessary and may or may not become permanent members. As a particular project gets into its later stages, usually past the priority phase, the committee may decide that line managers and supervisors from the user areas directly affected by the project should become ad hoc or advisory attendees of the committee meetings.

For example, a hospital might establish a steering committee composed of the CEO, a member of the medical staff, the chief financial officer, the CCRM, and a trustee with strong CR user experience. If the committee is recommending automation of the laboratory, the chief of pathology and the chief laboratory technologist might be asked to become ad hoc representatives until the project has been concluded.

The Mission

The primary mission of the computer resource steering committee is to ensure that the direction and usage of computer resources agree with the organization's strategic business plan. To this end, the committee recommends and maintains a long-range computer resources plan (discussed in Chapter 8).

The committee will establish priorities and direction for the CCRM. As users become more sophisticated, there is usually an increase in project requests. The central CR staff cannot satisfy all of these requests and, without the committee, will frequently be under pressure to supply all computer resources. Alternative recommendations for utilization of CR staff and budgets, along with the potential dollar savings and service, are presented by the CCRM for the committee's evaluation and selection. Those projects selected by the committee are given priority according to funding, staff availability, payback, and organizational goals.

Ranking of the major CR projects by the committee is necessary because of the numerous allocations possible for the CR staff and budgets. The committee representatives should be capable of putting into perspective their department goals versus the organization's goals. After projects are ranked, the committee member who represents a department with a high-priority application can act as a liaison with the CCRM and is responsible for ensuring the appropriate commitment and interaction through the UCRM.

Organizations selecting multiuser computer applications may have the committee participate in the vendor and software selection process. Some organizations limit the responsibility of the steering committee over the selection and control of all computer resources to an advisory role and sounding board. In other organizations, the committee might be a major committee, and all capital computer resource requests, including staff needs, might first have to undergo committee review and receive recommendation. In any case, the mission of the committee and the role of each of the members should be made clear and agreed upon from the outset.

Education

Ideally, steering committee members should have been exposed to previous usage of computer resources, either through educational or experiential backgrounds. They must be versed in their individual end-user objectives and must also understand the overall organizational goals and needs. Steering committee members must be familiar with the use of computers in organizations and with the basics of information systems theory. They must also recognize the potential for computer resources and services in the organization. In short, the members of the steering committee should possess the best available blend of experiential and academic knowledge.

Given the need for this expertise, the committee members should not delegate these responsibilities to junior members of their staff. For the committee to serve its mission, it must have the commitment and personal involvement of each member. It is the responsibility of the chairperson to see that the members maintain the committee's purpose, to educate and update members, and to be sure that they do not digress from their assigned roles.

Cautions

Not all organizations endorse a computer resource steering committee. A committee must not be set up to manage the central CR staff, nor is the steering committee the channel through which the CCRM reports. The CCRM reports to the CEO or COO, not to the steering committee.

Further, the committee should not be involved in the details of the central CR function. For instance, it should not determine whether additional memory is required or what model disk is best for a specific CR situation. However, the justification for this capital equipment is certainly within the role of the committee. The roles of the CCRM and of the steering committee must be clearly delineated. The chairperson must keep the committee within its scope of responsibility.

Some committees do not function because of individual members who do not always present the needs of the users whom they supposedly represent. The CR selection and implementation process can be hindered by one committee member directing the committee in a direction that is self-serving and not representative of the needs of the organization or the individual users. Systems projects will fail when applications and computer resources are forced upon users without prior knowledge or recommendation input.

If people with limited decision-making responsibility are on the committee, they may not have the ability to respond appropriately for the areas that they represent. Thus, user department conflicts can occur after a committee decision or recommendation has been made.

The self-interest of members may make it difficult for the committee to arrive at a consensus of what is best for the overall organization. Trying to get the committee to make a decision may be futile, or the final decision may reflect only the interests of the "strongest" member. This and other factors may cause an extended amount of time to pass without a decision or recommendation. The CEO or COO who feels that a decision should have been made may not wait, preempting the recommendations of the committee.

In a similar manner, these committees sometimes actually do address concerns that are not their responsibility. Valuable time may be wasted by studying areas not within the committee's scope. An example may be addressing the implementation process of an application or financial funding concerns.

These potential problems may dictate an approach where decisions concerning computer resources are made solely by the CEO or the COO and the CCRM. Before using the steering committee approach, the possible pitfalls should be recognized and addressed. It should be clear that the selection of the right people for the committee is of the utmost importance in this process.

Using the steering committee approach is a means of providing end-user interaction and can produce a synergistic effect that results in greater commitment from both the users and the CR staff. This effect can be enhanced by users participating in all phases of strategic planning and systems development. It will result in the removal of the systems mystique for users and will promote an understanding of and concern for the present and future success of computer resources.

The Agenda

The agenda of a meeting is set depending on the needs of each organization. Items such as the minutes of the last meeting are always necessary, and there must be time for open discussion. In addition, there are items that must be presented to the committee at least annually.

The computer resource cost to the organization can be reviewed annually by the committee. The computer resource plan must also be reviewed and approved annually. With the status of today's information and staffing demands on the health-care environment, it is important to confirm that the organization's business plan is being addressed by the computer resource plan. In addition, an annual update of applications and their status must be presented by the CCRM.

Other examples of a meeting agenda may include a specific meeting to discuss and establish priorities based on a list of identified application needs. The presentation of capital equipment computer requests by users may be an agenda item. For example, a user presenter may be required by

Figure 2-2. Needs and selection phase: the steering committee.

Members	Functions
Nursing Staff	Represent Users
Fiscal Staff	Prioritize Applications
Clinical Staff	Select Vendor(s)
Medical Staff	
Trustees	
Administration	
Computer Resources Staff	

the committee to justify a request in line with the organization's strategic business plan. Another agenda might include the review and approval of a request for proposal before it is sent to vendors.

The Development of a Computer Resource Steering Committee

One might look at the development of a computer resource steering committee as a two-phase process. The first stage is when an organization decides to pursue computer resources as part of their strategic business plan. In this case, the steering committee may be formed and given an initial responsibility of representing users, prioritizing applications, and selecting vendors, as previously discussed. Figure 2-2 shows a computer resource steering committee membership as formed to define computer resource needs and select appropriate vendors and applications.

Once this committee has been functioning and is looked upon by the organization as a standing committee, it can be considered ready for its second phase. This phase is the ongoing committee. In phase 2, the committee's responsibilities certainly include those in phase 1, but are now more general as the committee functions in a planning and monitoring process (Fig. 2-3). Chapter 9, "Diary of an Integrated Computer Resource," describes how one organization advanced through the two phases of development.

Conclusions

Two computer resource managers were identified. The user CR manager (UCRM) is the user area's advocate regarding computer resources. The UCRM is responsible for coordinating, with the CCRM, the use of the

Figure 2-3. Functions of the ongoing steering committee.

1. Provides representation for all areas
2. Provides adequate financial support
3. Sets major priorities
4. Communicates resource effectiveness
5. Promotes new applications
6. Monitors user satisfaction levels

end-user's computer resources and services, as well as managing the use and maintenance of the specific user applications. This person maintains the current computer resources and services and coordinates necessary enhancements and procedures. The UCRM must have both academic and experiential background in the use of computer resources.

The central CR manager (CCRM) must be as much at ease in the world of the users as in the role of a senior manager and in the specialized realm of technology. The organization's strategic business plan must be the focus of the organization's usage of computer resources, and it must be the CCRM who plans and maintains this direction. This manager faces the task of revising and replacing existing systems to reflect changes in both technology and organizational needs. This demanding position must be filled by a person who has a firm understanding of the overall organizational goals and who is committed to assisting users in meeting these goals. The CCRM must also possess a genuine sensitivity to users' needs, a balance of technical and managerial skills, and systems and planning orientation. In addition, the CCRM is primarily responsible for creating the environment to allow and foster interaction.

The computer resources steering committee is an organizational tool for maintaining continued interaction, cooperation, and joint user and CCRM accountability. It should be an interdisciplinary committee representing the necessary background and policies of the organization. The formation of a steering committee is essential to ensure adequate computer resource financing, organizational recognition, and an appropriate planning process. The direction of the committee must be to carry out the organization's strategic business plan through the use of computer resources. The committee should approve the CR long-range plan and priorities as it addresses the business plan. Six to eight senior mangers and ad hoc members (as deemed necessary) regulate CR use by assigning priorities to computer resource requests and by giving direction to the use of a central CR staff.

Questions

1. At a local visiting nurse association (VNA), the central CR manager is the comptroller. She has a bachelor's degree in Accounting and had worked for five years as a CPA before being employed as the comptroller. As the president of the VNA, what would you do to assure yourself that you had the most appropriate person serving as the CCRM?
2. Suppose that you are the UCRM of a department in a large hospital. You realize that a microcomputer would be a useful and low-cost resource for performing a task that is specific to your department and your department alone. Evaluating the effect of different fund-raising techniques on contributions might fall into this category of tasks. How do you convince the computer resource steering committee that this is an appropriate strategy for your department?
3. Suppose that you are on the computer resource steering committee for your organization. The chief of radiology has just been notified that the committee turned down his pet project, automation of the transcription section. How do you think the doctor will satisfy his CR needs? What can you do to head off potential problems?

Suggested Readings

Austin, C.J. 1988. *Information systems for health services.* 3rd ed. Ann Arbor, MI: Health Administration Press.

Goldberg, A.J., and R.A. DeNoble. 1986. Hospital Department Profiles. Chicago, IL: American Hospital Publishing, Inc.

Packer, C.L. February 20, 1988. Information management: CIOs have limited say in business planning. *Hospitals.*

Rockart, J.F. April 1982. The changing role of the information systems executive: a critical success factors perspective. Center for information systems research WP#85. Sloan School of Management. Cambridge, MA: Massachusetts Institute of Technology.

Rydell, R.L. Winter 1988. Organizing information management team at Baystate Health Systems. *Journal of Healthcare Information Management and Systems Society* 2(1).

Sneider, R.M. 1987. *Management guide to healthcare information systems.* Rockville, MD: Aspen Publishers.

CHAPTER 3

Strategies to Promote and Maintain Computer Resources

Introduction

Minicase 1: Absence of Interaction

The manager of a cancer registry bought a microcomputer and accompanying software applications to create and maintain a patient database, provide population statistics, and generate follow-up letters and address labels. The registry manager selected and purchased the microcomputer and software using no specific evaluation method other than his knowledge that other registry managers had microcomputers and frequently talked about how easy they were to use and what time-savers they were. The registry manager took no time to consider microcomputer management issues or to understand the various modes of microcomputer and software operation.

From the day the microcomputer was installed by the vendor, the staff continually complained that they did not have enough training on how the computer worked. They continually blamed the computer for letters being sent late to physicians and for their backlog of work. The manager believed that the software sold by the vendor was inadequate and different from that of other registries. Assistance was requested from the central computer resource (CR) department, but help was slow in coming because the department was not familiar with the software purchased and was trying to understand both the department's information need and how the software functioned. In summary, the cancer registry department was in over its head with automation and felt frustrated and misled.

Minicase 2: Presence of Interaction

A computer resource steering committee approved a request from the medical record department for a central medical record index system to retrieve patient demographic data and store the history of previous visits. The medical record supervisor participated in the selection of the software, and her staff now fully utilize the system's unique routines. Whenever there are problems that the supervisor cannot solve, she works side-by-side with the central CR analyst to troubleshoot and correct the problems. The supervisor exhibits a high level of satisfaction with the new system.

Discussion

The foregoing scenarios were both played out in the same organization. Why is one supervisor satisfied with the computer resources and the other frustrated and complaining? The answer may be found in the absence or presence of *interaction*. The cancer registry manager did not prepare himself properly for the installation; he believed that the software would be easy to use and that the central CR staff should be responsible for setting up the system. He would only operate it. The manager took little initiative in understanding the responsibilities of managing microcomputers and how the computer routines could be incorporated into the department's operation. The manager did not understand the computer's potential and pitfalls. The manager had no approach to system planning and offered only negative comment as to why the microcomputer would not work.

The medical records supervisor "took the bull by the horns" from the start and proceeded to examine closely the goals of the department and how computerization could assist in meeting those goals. She made visits to other organizations, took a computer course at a local college, did literature reviews, and generally made an all-out effort to become an expert on the new system. She realized that, if the system was to be her responsibility, she would need to be deeply involved in the planning, installation, and training phases, so that she could eventually be independent of vendor and CR department assistance. She worked side by side with the CR analyst. By troubleshooting problems and discussing hardware, software, and procedural concerns, she gained valuable insight into the system's capabilities, operation, and limitations.

No Simple Explanation

Organizations pay highly for consultants to answer their computer questions on how to design, improve, and implement methods to serve their computer needs. Administrators, physicians, and ancillary staff request that the answers not be in "computerese," but in simple language that explains how to plan and maintain an effective computer system.

There is no simple explanation. The only way to develop an effective computer system is for the CR staff to understand more about the user area than is found in just the required reports. Likewise, the end-user must understand the central CR staff's role and not simply expect CR personnel to be experts at mental telepathy who, through a combination of intuition, magic, and mind projection, always know the user department's needs with infinite precision.

Unstructured Involvement

Many users willingly commit themselves to unstructured and misunderstood involvement. This means that they understand that they must attend committee meetings and approve numerous memos and reports that define and plan their systems. Furthermore, they believe that the CR staff will be responsible for all of the system's planning, training, and implementation and that the end-user will only assume responsibility for the acceptance or rejection of the final product. By the same token, to the CR staff, user involvement often means working in a rather mechanical manner, literally developing what is requested rather than what is needed or usable. The CR staff sets up the system and the end-user approves the final product; however, this type of involvement does not work.

Unstructured involvement results in the central CR area spending many hours and dollars on projects that are never used. Useless system features result because the CR staff prepared specifications by the "letter of the law" rather than the "spirit of the law." Projects can seemingly last forever as users attempt to define and redefine exactly what they want the system to do and CR staff obediently redefine the additional, forgotten, or misunderstood changes.

Active Interaction

If unstructured and passive involvement does not ensure a successful system, how then do users arrive at a meaningful, workable system? One method that works, the method that is proposed to both users and CR staff, is active interaction.

Interaction can ensure a continuous and effective relationship between the central CR and user staffs. Interaction means that the end-user wears a systems analyst hat and that the CR staff communicates in the end-user's language and asks intelligent questions. Interaction means a complete team approach—the sharing of system analysis responsibility (beginning with project initiation and continuing through implementation), the use of interdepartmental controls, and the sharing of the resulting accolades. Interaction ensures ongoing interdepartmental dialogue.

Who takes the initiative in the interaction process? Ideally, interaction occurs when the end-user and the CR staff independently assume the responsibility to develop interaction techniques. Both must commit themselves to a successful project regardless of the other's degree of involvement. Active interaction is like a successful marriage in which both partners are willing to give more than they receive.

Education

One approach that is valuable as a first step in interaction is education in a formal setting. Staff should be encouraged to attend seminars on the use of computers. Local colleges offer courses that provide an introduction to data processing. These courses will introduce one to the responsibilities involved in using computer resources. A formal computer education course can remove the mystique of computers and enlighten users as to its potential.

The central CR staff can also make available formal computer training courses for end-users. A comprehensive computer course will be enlightening to both user and CR personnel. The CR instructor will recognize the concerns of users and can put many fears and misconceptions to rest, and an in-house course will help to promote interdepartmental dialogue. Figure 4-2 in Chapter 4 is a sample in-house computer course agenda.

Visiting Each Other's Workplace

The importance of face-to-face interaction and on-site activities cannot be overemphasized. Many misunderstandings develop when individuals have no concrete idea of the basic elements of an area's operation. Many organizational procedures are defined by space limitations and equipment needs. Although formal education is the first step in real communication, nothing can substitute for the experience of seeing and touching the real thing. Users might hear the terms line printer or CPU (central processing unit), but these items of hardware become real only when actually viewed in operation.

Members of the user staff should ask to visit the central CR areas. The CR staff can also take the initiative by extending invitations for tours of the CR areas. Often users "throw the data over the fence and the reports are thrown back" with no idea as to what happens regarding program logic and computer operations.

A technique that works well when explaining why users should enter data into the computer in their area is to have one user become the data entry operator using the user's own source documents. The user can see firsthand what happens when nonuser staff try to enter illegible or incomplete data into the computer. The reasons for user self-entry become obvious. The tour of the CR area should include a demonstration of the printing of end-user reports. This demonstration will reveal the time and preparation needed before reports can be delivered. Many people believe that the computer works with the "speed of light" and that five-page statistical reports for 100 diagnoses can be printed instantly. An actual demonstration of report preparation brings CR responsibility into focus for the users. The time-consuming decollating and bursting necessary before a report can be delivered demonstrates the reality of data processing and eliminates the myth of simply "pushing a button."

The user area should reciprocate and invite CR personnel to tour the user area to learn why various input and output routines are needed. When viewing the laboratory, for example, CR staff can realize the time involved and the knowledge necessary to obtain data prior to terminal input. Discussing with CR personnel the nature of laboratory reports used by physicians will prove the usefulness of the information. If the central CR staff has an understanding of the user area, the importance of maintaining computer response and uptimes and of fast turnaround of broken terminals and printers will become clear.

An expanded version of an end-user area tour is to assign a CR staff member to the user area temporarily. The CR person can be given responsibility to perform certain tasks for the end-user. This person will develop a working dialogue with end-user personnel and thus come to understand the user's work requirements.

Strategy Sessions

It is vital that interaction take place before important committee meetings and planning sessions. When CR staff and user staff get together, they can work out an agenda and discuss the items to be presented. This provides an opportunity to review the appropriate data and reports and the manner in which they are interpreted. Preparation in an informal setting allows for brainstorming and an exchange of ideas that might be considered out of place in a full committee setting. Differing points of view and areas of concern of each specialty become apparent and can be accommodated and reconciled to the goals of the group. The end result of these sessions will be formal meetings that run more smoothly and accomplish more objectives. In addition, the parties involved will be more aware of each other's thoughts regarding the optimal operation of the user area.

Attending User Meetings

CR staff should frequently attend user committee meetings. If the CR staff understands how systems are to be used, it can assist more effectively in the definition of application features by being able to "read between the lines" when screens are defined.

It is important that both CR and user personnel understand the methods used to produce sophisticated statistical reports. For example, in order for a cancer committee to use relative survival rates, it is necessary for the committee and the CR analyst to understand an actuarial table and the standard error of the mean in relationship to the statistic. This understanding will lead to more accurate presentation of the data.

Physician committee members can contribute valuable insight into the interpretation of data because of their clinical experience and their knowledge of the current medical literature. CR staff can offer fresh insight into or a simple solution to a problem because they have an impartial view of the situation. For example, at one cancer committee meeting, data on the treatment of cancer of the prostate were presented. The physicians were able to point out that reports presenting these data should not include transurethral resection (TUR) because it is a diagnostic or palliative procedure and not a treatment. To eliminate this category, however, would be to throw away valuable information. The CR analyst suggested the simple compromise of listing the category as "TUR ONLY." Thus, the data were provided in the report, with the medically correct interpretation and emphasis. The committee's input kept the report medically appropriate; the CR analyst's input kept the data complete.

Flow Chart and Systems Design

User and CR staff should integrate their needs for system features. Instead of the user orally explaining what the feature should be, the feature's format should be put on paper. Discussions aided by a visual document can be better understood by both parties. In addition, the user should demonstrate the logic that will go into the feature through the use of a flow chart.

CR personnel should discuss the requested feature before a draft is initiated, but again the draft should be made by the end-user area. Vendor selection or programming should not begin until the requests are formatted and the logic is defined by the end-user.

Even small changes in data needs and reports can have major implications for a computer system. Therefore, it is vital that both the end-user and the central CR analyst decide whether a change is sufficiently important (i.e., medically appropriate) to warrant "tinkering" with the system. This aspect of interaction takes into account the amount of work necessary to make the change and will ensure the integrity of the data and of reports over time.

Draft specifications were historically prepared by the CR analyst. This resulted in reports and screens looking the way the analyst thought they should look. Having the end-user design screens and reports results in a more usable end product. Undoubtedly, there will be changes in the initial designs and the CR analyst will make suggestions for the logic and reporting formats, but the user personnel should feel comfortable with the resulting output.

Use of Prototypes

Detailed system specifications can have their limits. Planning a carefully thought-out system and then maintaining its design during actual implementation is difficult, if not impossible, to do in one pass. Many times the user cannot visualize how a system will operate in its final and most effective state. It is the actual hands-on experience of manipulating data during entry, retrieval, and reporting that provides a thorough understanding of what is really desired and a system's possible limitations.

Installing a computer model and allowing the user to "play" with it can be a very effective technique. Prototype heuristic approaches allow users to arrive at a workable and understandable system, provide confidence in the system, and speed up the training and implementation process.

Test Data and Calculations

When it is time to test the system, the end-user staff should be responsible for supplying sample data. In addition, sample calculations should be manually prepared by user personnel and used to verify the accuracy of the test report or screen format. If the CR analyst provides the test data, the analyst will check only what appears reasonable from the CR perspective. The analyst does not have the end-user's background and specialized knowledge and cannot be aware of all data input possibilities. The personnel of the user staff are the experts in the usage of the reports or screens and therefore should confirm the features' accuracy and reasonableness. Items such as edit checks for data being entered should include test data for all input possibilities and potential errors. This interaction will provide good, solid screen formats and reporting, rather than well-programmed but unreliable information.

Documentation

The end-user staff should prepare all systems manuals and user documents explaining computer systems developed both in-house and by software vendors. The CR analyst can then verify the documentation and reconcile system differences with the end-user.

For vendor-provided software, it is the responsibility of the vendor to furnish the system documentation. However, it is necessary for users to convert this documentation into procedure manuals for the people working with the system on a day-by-day basis. Vendor-provided manuals are often all-encompassing, and most users need only selected instructions for dealing with their unique needs. For example, a transcriptionist in radiology would need documentation for only a limited amount of features.

Having the end-user design the systems documentation ensures that at least one person from each area understands the system's functions. Without such an approach, the CR analyst will be the only expert on the system. System documentation ensures that the painstaking efforts of all involved will be permanent and will transcend personnel changes in either area. Users must also tailor their documentation to accommodate any custom programming.

Minicase 3: CR Department Interprets Payroll Policy

A good example of a situation in which an improper approach to documentation caused a problem is the implementation of a payroll system in a home health agency. A work committee that included the payroll supervisor was formed. The payroll department had never documented its present operation and thus had no perception of the complete payroll system. It was left to the system analyst to determine present procedures, workflow, and output. The payroll supervisor reviewed the written systems definition and even signed off on the proposed system, but the supervisor did not take time for the extensive interaction and commitment necessary for such a large scale system and was not prepared to assume the responsibility for a user manual.

During the first year of the payroll operation, there were many calls to the CR department for clarification of the operation of the system. Requests for clarification of system procedures were made routinely. How were calculations made? How were deductions determined? The CR department was perceived as the payroll expert, and often payroll policy was interpreted by them. As turnover occurred in the payroll area, the payroll department became more heavily dependent on the CR department for training its clerks—all because the supervisor had only a cursory understanding of the payroll system's operation and had made no commitment to develop an in-depth understanding of the system through the preparation and maintenance of a user manual.

Discussion

The foregoing situation could have been avoided through interaction. If the payroll supervisor had been held responsible for a user manual, the supervisor would have become intimately involved in the system's design and installation and would have been forced to know the limits and extent of the system's operation. Moreover, if the user manual had been prepared by the payroll supervisor, the CR department could have verified the documentation and reconciled system differences with the supervisor. A user-prepared manual can reveal differences of opinions and misunderstandings regarding procedures, functions, and limits, and these differences can be readily corrected or discussed. Discussing these differences would have educated the analyst and the supervisor and led to program and procedure changes that would have further enhanced the operation and usefulness of the overall system.

Controlling Data and Reports

The end-user staff should monitor real-time entry procedures to maintain the integrity of the data being collected. This may mean periodically reentering data from the same source documents and determining a percentage of accuracy. Controls for a storeroom inventory system may be as simple as the unit count of items issued. Storeroom and user personnel can use this total to ensure complete processing of the data. Without such control the end-user cannot ensure the accurate processing of data. Considering the inventory decisions based on computer-generated data, it is essential that data input be as accurate as possible.

The output reports and screens should be checked for reasonableness, and "pulse points" should be developed. A "pulse point" in the storeroom would be the inventory turnover statistic, which is reviewed for reasonableness and effectiveness.

Parallel Systems

Whenever system changes or "improvements" in existing screens and reports are implemented, it is important to consider maintaining a comparison system for a limited period. The end-user must compare the present system with the new system to ensure that changes have been made successfully. Often, what appears to be a small system change can have a significant and costly effect on the total system. The uniqueness of many computer programs can lead to unexpected problems if new systems are not verified before they are implemented.

For some systems it is not feasible to operate an extensive parallel system. The response time and complexity of a real-time system may make it unreasonable for the end-user to duplicate input and hardware in an attempt to develop a parallel system. In this situation, the CR staff may develop duplicate sets of application programs, using one set for the live system and the other for testing enhancements. When a change in the test computer system has been approved by both user and CR staff, the change can be made in the live system.

For example, when making a change in a radiology order entry system that will require that the last test date be printed on a service request form, the new program change may be tried by the user in a test system to determine whether the change was made properly. The test will also ensure that other features of the system were not affected. Once the change is determined to be acceptable, the new print program can be transferred to the live system.

One method for teaching users to understand real-time computer system concepts is to create test master files for user training. For example, nurses can learn to order patient services by accessing a fictitious patient and then entering services as if the patient was real. The system will simulate the actual ordering functions and perform all VDT lead-throughs without actually updating live files. This method can also be used for ongoing training of new employees.

Interdepartmental Communications

The user and the central CR staff should meet periodically to review the relationship between the areas. These can be formal meetings, or they can be social occasions centered around coffee or lunch. In either case, continual dialogue between the areas will serve to promote cooperation.

Improved communications result when the end-user puts all requests for CR services in writing. Written requests commit the end-user. Hallway conversations that result in immediate action by CR personnel often are frustrating for the CR staff; the user may simply be asking "can you?" when the CR employee hears a "must have" request. Committing a request to writing encourages the user to reflect on all of the variables involved.

Troubleshooting

Troubleshooting plays an important part in the process of interaction. The CR staff must quickly respond to and rectify problems that occur in the end-user's system. Because user staff have been involved in the development of the system from the outset, their knowledge will help focus attention on specific problem areas and save system analyst time. Instead of saying "I don't know what is wrong with this report," an educated user might be able to tell the CR analyst, "I think the wrong group of patients is being extracted."

Work Committee

A successful computer system must have both the support and the participation of the people who will be responsible for using and maintaining it. Work committee members are those supervisors and user computer resource managers with day-to-day responsibility and hands-on experience with the computer system. The committee promotes participation and accountability for the success or failure of the system. Chapter 6 details a work committee assignment.

The committee can be chaired by the person most responsible for the day-to-day operations of the system (if the system operates generally within one area). The committee should meet at least monthly to bring each member up to date on individual responsibilities. Senior management should attend such committee meetings by special invitation only so as not to stifle frank discussions, which are encouraged.

Continuing Interaction

The end-user can invite CR personnel to a local, regional, or national allied meeting. Discussions with people from other organizations will provide CR staff with insight into user needs and concerns. As a result of federal and state legislation, most users are now being forced to consider opportunities for computer applications, and all parties can benefit from extended dialogue.

CR and user staff should participate together in post-implementation cost-benefit studies and continually learn from the experiences gained through follow-up studies. These studies will often reveal benefits not evident in the feasibility study, as well as the absence of benefits that were expected. Investigation of unrealized benefits may reveal deficiencies in training or implementation methods or lack of understanding of the end-user's operation. Once these deficiencies are recognized, the expected benefits can be achieved. This knowledge educates the CR and user staffs for future studies and can even generate new, feasible studies for additional projects. The bottom line is that, through these studies, the presence of computer resources is justified, the efforts of user staff are justified, and recognition is given to the user and the CR staff for a job well done.

Each area can assist the other in gaining understanding of their respective needs by swapping journal articles. When an article appears in a national journal describing the use of a particular system, it should be read by personnel from both areas. This review provides ongoing education and may generate ideas for additional system features.

Publications

A successful computer installation should be made known to other users. This can be accomplished through the writing of articles explaining the effort and the techniques that were used in the development process. The articles should be coauthored by user personnel and CR staff. Publications play an important part in helping to maintain the quality of a computer system. Published articles document the process that defines the technical procedures and output resulting from successful interaction and instill in the coauthors a sense of responsibility and a feeling of shared success. Most important, publications given credit where credit is due, and no one feels left out or resentful if the accolades and attention are appropriately shared. This type of interaction brings pride to end-user areas and individuals, is good public relations for the organization, and gives the public confidence in the application.

Senior Management Interaction

Much as been written about the need for senior management support of users and CR supervisors who are developing computer systems. Part of this support rests in the realization that some of the already-discussed interaction techniques may require extensive time of user supervisors. Senior management may need to authorize temporary user staff or overtime during computer installations. For example, the installation of an inventory system with vendor and item profiles may require that a temporary or contract person be hired for a few months to relieve the supervisor or staff of duties that cannot be properly handled during installation.

Evolution of a Conditional Computer System

In the past, users "signed off" on a system's design after the CR staff prepared reports based on what both parties perceived to be the user's needs. In reality, however, the users generally could not, and would not, stay within this defined "contract." Interaction techniques and prototype development are approaches that deal with this "breach of contract" problem.

There is another phenomenon for user and CR supervisors to consider in their quest for the "perfect" CR (Priest and O'Sullivan 1983). Individuals involved in a system's development must understand that development is a dynamic process. There is an underlying concept that both user and CR staff must grasp: let it be called the "evolution of a conditional CR." The process of implementing a CR is an evolution because it is a stepwise movement toward a goal, a movement in which each step is determined in part by what has preceded it. The term "conditional" is used because a CR can only be "perfect" for a particular point in time and must be capable of changing in response to the users' needs and changing perspective of the system.

As illustrated in Figure 3-1, a computer system is time-dependent on a user's current experience, perspective, and position within the organization. Starting at point A, CR features are determined by a participant's perspective at that time. With the experience gained and the sophistication developed in using the system, new features (B) become necessary. This cumulative knowledge will in turn help both user and CR personnel progress to a point where more (or fewer) features (C) are essential. Thus, the system will evolve and change in a pattern that is conditional on the knowledge and perspective of the individuals involved in the project at particular times. The challenge for all participants is to recognize and work within this conditional evolutionary framework.

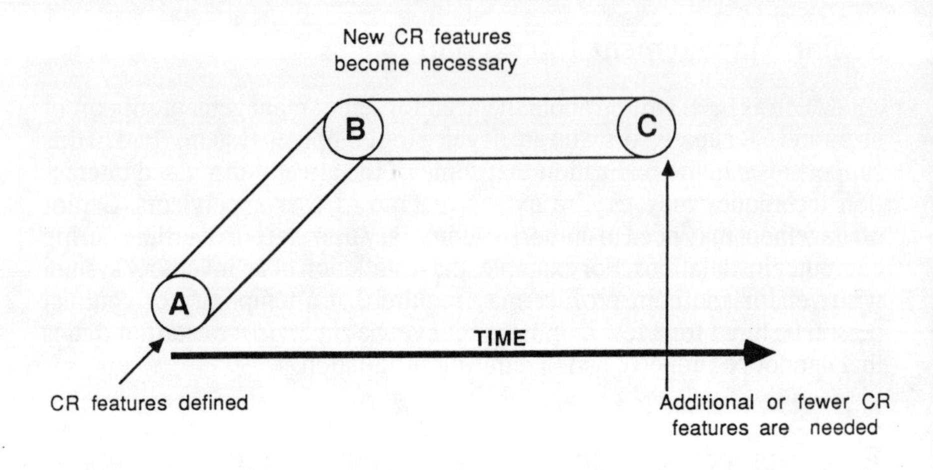

Figure 3-1. The evolution of a conditional computer resource. Reprinted from *The Health Care Supervisor*, Vol. 1, No. 4, July, 1983, p. 89, with permission of Aspen Publishers, Inc.

Minicase 4: An Evolutionary Example

An example will help to explain this concept. An organization has made a commitment to install a real-time patient registration system and put together a request for proposal detailing desired system features for vendor bids. These desired features are the result of the organization's understanding of its current system, its deficiencies, and the manner in which a real-time, state of the art registration system will fit into existing operation and policies. The organization is now at point A.

After the system is installed and in use, the individuals involved develop a different perspective of the registration process. They can see that a patient history and demographic information is easily retrieved and controlled; the real-time system incorporates checks and "pulse points" that in the past were purely organizational in nature. At this point, B, the organization realizes that the central registration concept (in which all patients are registered in a specific location before receiving ancillary, nursing, or physician services) is slowing the delivery of services to patients. The real-time system makes it efficient and practical to have physician offices schedule their patients directly into the computer via telecommunications. The patient can report directly to the ancillary department for service, bypassing the registration department. Without the experience of using the system over time, this step would have been difficult to envision.

By distributing the registration function, the organization can expect to move on to point C, at which the ancillary departments will ask for new system features as their experience with the system grows. The message to CR and user supervisors in this and other cases is that the supervisors must step back and regard what they expect to be a "perfect" CR. Both must realize that new opportunities will exist and that the system will evolve with the experience and perspective gained by actual operation. These opportunities are contingent on what has happened previously and must be managed in light of the "evolution."

Changing the Conditional CR

Many of the required procedural changes and uses that accompany a new system require an adjustment period for the users before the full effect of the system can be evaluated. A period of time is usually required for the user staff to integrate fully the new features with standard operating procedures. During this adjustment period, there may be a minimum of feature changes allowed by the CR management (except for errors) until the system has been fully installed and used. Once the effect of the system and new procedures is understood, then the end-user can discuss and request changes through the interaction technique of requiring requests to be written. A reasonable adjustment before changes would be made may be three to six months.

A realistic compromise concerning immediate system changes can usually be made between the user and CR areas. The CR staff can make available a fixed number of staff hours for essential system changes within the first month of installation. Thus, the end-user area will have a set number of CR staff hours available and can determine how those hours should be allocated while still allowing the CR supervisor to remain on schedule with other CR projects. Once the allotted hours are used, the period of adjustment must be accepted (or else another compromise with the CR supervisor must be made.

Conclusion

The interaction techniques discussed in this chapter are summarized in Table 3-1. When the staff of one area put themselves in the shoes of another area, they develop an appreciation of each other's concerns. Open and candid dialogue is promoted, and the end result is a workable computer system.

Table 3-1. Techniques that promote interaction between user and CR staff.

User Staff	CR Staff
1. Taking the initiative to promote interaction	1. Taking the initiative to promote interaction
2. Receiving instruction in computer concepts	2. Teaching basic computer concepts to users.
3. Asking to review the CRs area; inviting CR staff to review the user area	3. Asking to review the user area; inviting users to review the CRs area
4. Inviting CR staff to a user committee meeting at which a computer–prepared report is to be presented.	4. Asking to attend a committee meeting at which a computer report is to be presented.
5. Drafting the design of a report with CR assistance; preparing a flow chart of logic; designing the system first on paper	5. Offering to assist the users in designing reports and the system's logic; doing no coding and not obtaining quotations from software vendors until the system or report is designed.
6. Providing and entering test data for new or changed reports; doing manual calculations and comparing with computer report	6. Having the user provide the data and manual calculations using test data.
7. Insisting on preparing the system manual that documents and explains the computer system	7. Having the user staff prepare the systems manual that describes the computer system.
8. Controlling real–time monitoring of all output reports; developing pulse points	8. Monitoring control totals and pulse points
9. Making all requests to CRs in writing	9. Requiring that report and application requests be in writing
10. "Playing with" a prototype, its system, and its entry, retrieval, and report routines	10. Installing a prototype so the user can play with entry, retrieval, and report routines
11. Checking parallel runs for all system acceptance	11. Having the user check parallel runs for all changes
12. Periodically meeting with CR staff to review relationships between staffs	12. Periodically meeting with the user staff to show CR willingness to meet user needs and concerns
13. Inviting CR staff to a user association meeting	13. Asking to attend user association meetings
14. Sending articles on user systems to the CR for review and education	14. Sending CR articles on user systems to the user staff for review and education
15. Training a CR analyst in user functions	15. Assigning a CR analyst to the user area to learn system procedures
16. Writing an article and including CR staff as coauthor	16. Writing an article and including the user as coauthor.

Reprinted from *The Health Care Supervisor*, volume 1, number 4, July 1983, pages 93–94, with permission of Aspen Publishers, Inc.

The implementation of a computer system is a dynamic, not a static, process. The end-user staff must actively interact with the CR staff if the full potential of the system is to be realized. In the past, it may have been productive for a computer resources area to install a system and walk away, performing only required maintenance. Modern management information systems, however, have a great deal of flexibility and offer a wide range of possibilities. Management of these systems that does not include user interaction and that does not envision the ongoing development of the system will negate much of this potential.

A primary benefit of interaction among computer resources and end-user staff, physician, patient, and community is effective computer reporting. This results when the people responsible for preparing and using the system are able to work effectively together and understand one another's concerns.

A central CR manager once commented on how good a particular user's computer system was. The user's response was, "It should be good—you made me do half the work!" This is true interaction.

Questions and Assignments

1. The accounting and computer resource staff continually blame each other for problems involving the financial computer applications. The supervisor in patient accounting believes that the CR staff should be responsible for printing selected reports and notifying accounting far in advance when the computer will not be available. The CR manager believes that the patient accounting staff is not being reasonably sensitive to computer resource staff and schedule responsibilities. You are the accounting manager. How do you get the different areas to work together to solve problems, rather than complain about the other's staff. You are the CR manager. How do you address this situation?

2. Most computer literacy courses are taught from the perspective of what the computer "expert" defines as computer literacy. Define computer literacy as perceived by the user. To do this, first survey two computer resource users and ask each to name five topics that should be part of a computer literacy course. Present their definitions in class using the blackboard and discuss the results.

Suggested Readings

Bullers, W.I., Jr., R.A. Reid, and H.L. Smith. October 1987. Negotiating the computer revolution: suggestions for health care supervisors. *The Healthcare Supervisor* 6(1): 44–57.

Lucas H.C., Jr. 1982. *Information systems concepts for management*. New York: McGraw–Hill Book Co.

Priest, S.L. 1982. *Managing hospital information systems*. Rockville, MD: Aspen Publishers.

Priest, S.L., and V.J. O'Sullivan. July 1983. The computer is coming—what should I do? *The Health Care Supervisor* 1(4): 75–94.

CHAPTER 4

Identifying Information Problems and Computer Resource Needs

Introduction

"We need a microcomputer! We need to buy this graphics package!" These comments are increasingly heard as current and potential users of computer resources seek to increase services and productivity through opportunities offered by advances in computer hardware and software technology. Computer technology can be the solution for users pressured with increased government reporting regulations and administrative demands for increased productivity and reporting and improved services, while at the same time being required to operate under constraints of cost and staffing budgets.

Before this technology is acquired, however, users must identify their information problems and needs and determine whether computerization will meet them. The identification of these needs usually determines what, if any, hardware and software are necessary.

The increased demand by users for timely, accurate, and sensitive information is forcing organizations to recognize the importance of information as an organizational resource and to recognize computer resources as a management tool that can be used to manage and monitor spiraling costs through improving user productivity. Finding methods to identify these potential computer resources to meet organizational information objectives is the challenge to innovative managers.

A Common Approach

One approach to computerization is to first acquire a computer, buy application packages, and then determine how they are to be used. This all-too-common approach has been used by many organizations and has all-too-frequently resulted in uncontrolled computer costs and disappointed users as the acquisitions do not meet expectations or require efforts not previously realized.

Some hardware and software requirements are determined solely through vendor recommendations. Sometimes an organization with little computer resource (CR) experience attempts to implement vendor-recommended packages that may not quite satisfy user needs. These packages in turn cause additional problems if users are required to conform to procedures that do not fit their area's method of operation and management style. Both frustration and disruption can result when unexpected, unacceptable, and unplanned changes are forced upon users. In essence, the user has to conform to computer and software specifications even though the changes may not be in the best interest of the organization.

Sometimes an organization with little or no experience in CR concepts may further complicate the problem by not understanding the time and methods necessary to implement CRs, and this may lead to dissatisfaction with CR utilization and implementation schedules because reality may differ from the vendor's promises of overnight delivery and immediate implementation. For instance, the CR may have been acquired on the vendor's promise that the systems could be installed in three weeks; meanwhile, the user staff is only half-trained and four weeks have already gone by. In addition, if the new application is replacing an existing service, there can be unacceptable costs because both the existing and the new service are being paid for simultaneously. These situations may result in pressure to complete the implementation according to the salesperson's promises, even though the proposed schedule may be unrealistic.

Minicase 1: Unrealistic CR Conversion Schedules

The aforementioned scenario actually happened. The mandate of an organization resulted in a rushed conversion from an outside vendor service to an on-site system. After the hurried six-month conversion, it was discovered that the organization's new accounts-receivable system was not operating properly. The software had not produced an accurate bill for two months because of a file conversion error not noticed during conversion. The user staff was too rushed to maintain adequate audit trails during the conversion of the receivables database. It was 12 months after conversion before the accounts-receivable system was as satisfactory as it had been before the conversion.

Another example of a less than successful attempt at installing computer resources is a home health agency that had four different computer vendors in two years. In each instance the agency management did not involve the users in the definition of needs and the software selection process. Senior management did not understand the detail of the user's needs and proceeded to select vendors and applications that had been successfully installed at other agencies without realizing that many agencies have different methods and policies for data input and output reporting. The changes in user procedures required to satisfy the needs of the new computer software could not be effectively absorbed by the staff because there had been no staff interaction and cooperation in the need definition and selection phases of implementation. In effect, the user had no idea how the CR could be used without complete disruption of the current processes. Each time a new vendor was selected, unrealistic deadlines were forced on the new vendor and the user was faced with inadequate time for systems planning and definition. Senior management still believes that the systems failures were the fault of each of the four computer vendors. Management did not look at the process that they used to select the vendors.

Selecting computer equipment and applications first and then determining how they will fit into the organization can cause user frustration, discord, and resistance. An approach that does not consider the needs and attitudes of the people who will use the system will have a less than effective outcome.

A method that has user participation, awareness, and cooperation as part of its process is one in which the organization's and the user's information needs and problems are recognized and defined first. Only after this first step can the software and computers be selected to fit the defined need.

Should a Consultant be Hired?

Should a consultant be hired to assist in determining needs and selecting computer resources? The answer depends on whether the organization has its own CR staff and the degree of experience possessed by users and the CR staff. If there is no CR experience within the organization, then an outside consultant is a prime consideration. The consultant will advise on decisions concerning applications, staff, equipment, process, and costs. The final selection decisions will still be made by the organization.

If the organization's staff lacks experience in areas such as hardware selection, then a consultant could be hired to guide the selection process with the staff performing the needs analysis. If political issues affect the selection process, such as when senior managers disagree on which areas should be addressed first, an outside consultant can often provide an unbiased opinion. Sometimes conditions in the organization may require a third party to reinforce an opinion, such as when a decision is not really clear and support is needed to remove any question of bias on the part of the decision-maker or -makers.

When considering the current status of CR services, an organization may want a consultant to provide an opinion on the current level of services. It may want an opinion on whether an on-site approach should be considered or whether the organization should use an outside vendor to provide services. In determining these consultant services, it is necessary to consider the degree of involvement of the consultant. Will the consultant carry out all phases of the project, such as long-range plans and recommendations, site visits, interviews, and the writing of a request for proposal (RFP), or should the consultant simply guide and advise the organization's staff? In addition, it must be determined at what phase of the project the consultant's services will no longer be needed.

Organizations may want their staff to be responsible for the day-to-day project tasks and to receive guidance from the consultant in order to better understand the selected systems. This experience will prove invaluable when the staff assumes responsibility for the implemented system at a later date. The staff will also be prepared to handle future projects without a need for further consultant services. It is important, however, to ensure that the on-site staff has the time necessary to accomplish both the additional workload and present system priorities.

Fees

Fees for a consultant vary. For an organization acquiring assistance in the selection of hardware and software, the fee will usually represent 1 to 3% of the five-year CR hardware and software cost. This cost is a minimal investment to provide objective input for a decision that may represent $50,000 to $500,000 annually.

Consultant's Bias

In selecting a consultant, one may want to learn whether this consultant always recommends the same vendor. Many consultants have limited experience and will tend to recommend the vendors with whom they feel the most comfortable. This may limit the opportunity to obtain what is best for a particular organization.

The CR Enthusiast

Caution should be taken when looking for CR experience within the organization. Use discretion when allowing a non-CR professional to choose your CR direction. Do not allow a computer enthusiast to put you in a position where he or she is the only person who knows your computer resources and you have a computer "just like" the one at the enthusiast's home. Business microcomputers and centrally managed computers are much different than one-person microcomputers used at home.

Enthusiasts are not consultants. Enthusiasts know a lot about computers, they love to share their knowledge, and they work long, hard hours to make computers do wonderful things. When all is said and done, however, the CR enthusiast will not be available when needed. You will be stuck with a very limited computer resource, and its application may not be exactly what is needed. The application may not be able to be changed by anyone other than the enthusiast, who is busy doing "his own job."

Which Consulting Firm Should Be Hired?

If the organization decides to hire outside assistance for hardware and software selection and contract negotiation, it should consider consulting only firms experienced in health-care systems. Consulting firms can be identified through one's peer associations such as the American Society of Healthcare Consultants, the College of American Pathologists (CAP), the Healthcare Financial Management Association (HFMA), and the American College of Healthcare Executives (ACHE). Telephone calls, letters, and informal conversations with associates will usually provide three or four firms that offer appropriate CR consulting services. These same associates will also reveal those firms that should not be considered.

Prior to contacting a firm, one should decide on the scope and needs of the computer resources and the reason for assistance. It must be clear whether the organization needs assistance in evaluation, recommendations, implementation, and/or follow-up. A firm should be required to respond to the organization's needs with a written proposal. The organization should schedule interviews with the people who will manage and carry out the project. The method in which the firm's written response is submitted should be specified in the request for proposal, and the proposal should be in the same format and include the same requirements for all firms.

It is most important to evaluate the consulting staff that will be assigned to the project, the people who will be doing the actual work. Hiring a prestigious consulting firm without considering the individuals involved in the project could result in the firm assigning persons with limited health-care and CR backgrounds. This could affect the length of the project and its degree of success or failure.

The firm's proposal should include detailed information on each prospective consultant. The proposal should address the prospective consultant's CR experience, listing organizations and projects to which they were previously assigned.

Further, the percentage of time that each consultant will be devoting to the project should be specified. Sometimes a firm may assign a consultant to many clients, and thus the consultant may not always be available for an immediate need of the organization. This should be considered when selecting a firm.

An organization that is seeking to hire a consultant to complement the on-site CR staff must specify the type of assistance being requested. For instance, if the organization's staff experience is limited to software evaluation, it may want a consultant who can lend hardware selection experience to the project. This need should be clearly presented in the RFP and should be understood by the consulting firm.

Before a firm is selected, a reference check should be made on each person to be assigned to the project. Preferably, these checks should be with comparable organizations that have previously used the individual's services. The reference check covers all aforementioned concerns regarding the consultants.

The firm's response should include fixed costs and expenses, the project methodology to be used by the consulting firm, the degree of participation that will be required of the organization's staff, and dates when the project can begin and be completed.

Table 4-1 is a sample evaluation matrix used to compare two consulting firms. The matrix was designed to fit this organization's particular needs. The organization thought that its staff was inexperienced in vendor hardware and software selection methods and therefore sought a consulting firm that could assist the CR staff in this area. In addition, the organization wanted its staff to acquire experience in the selection process and sought a firm that could provide guidance to the users as well as share day-to-day selection responsibilities. The matrix compares various selection criteria, costs, degree of responsibility to be assumed by the firm and by the organization's own staff, the experience of the to-be-assigned consultants, and the firm's estimate for project completion. A firm was chosen only after reference checks were made on both the firm and the consultants to be assigned to the organization, and extensive on-site interviews were held with each proposed consultant.

Table 4-1. Evaluation of consultants.[a]

	Consultant A	Consultant B
Fixed costs	$22,000	$27,000
Estimated expenses	5,500	1,300
**Total cost	$27,500	$28,300
	Planning	
Define present system	In-house staff to do most of work; document system, volumes, etc.	In-house staff to assist firm
Prepare long-range plan	Advise	Staff to assist
Prepare RFP	Major effort in-house	Firm B prepares RFP but in-house to assist
Hardware evaluation	In-house responsibility	Yes
Software evaluation	Yes	Yes
Vendor selection	Yes	Advise
Negotiations	Advise	Advise
Recommend staffing	Yes	Yes
Percentage of time consultant on project	1 day a week	3 days per week
	Consultant Experience	
Health-care experience	10 years—DP management	14 years—consulting
Real-time experience	Yes	Yes
Microcomputer experience	No	Yes
User background	No	Yes
Software experience	Limited	Yes
Contract Negotiations	Limited	Yes

Table 4-1, continued.

	Schedule	
Time	5–6 months	3–4 months

Summary:
1. Firm B will commit more staff than Firm A. Firm A expects much from our limited and inexperienced staff. Firm B brings their staff on site to handle day-to-day responsibilities. Our staff will closely assist firm B.
2. Firm A includes vendor selection. Firm B does not.

Recommendation: Due to comparable costs and the fact that Consultant B will assist with vendor selection, Consultant B is recommended. We will be getting more vendor assistance, and our staff will be given guidance and thus acquire experience useful when we assume total support responsibilities.

[a]Reprinted from *Managing Hospital Information Systems* by S. L. Priest, 1982, p. 35, with permission of Aspen Publishers, Inc.

User Education Sessions

The implementation of a CR can be complex and involve commitments from many people. If users are not ready for the CR or fear the implementation, then the CR is a candidate for failure.

The fears that some users have of computerization can often be reduced with an education program directed toward teaching the fundamentals of computers and CR capabilities and responsibilities. A user who can understand and is prepared for computerization will usually be committed to a successful CR and be ready to provide the interaction described in Chapter 3. Users who have a basic knowledge of computers and CRs help to recognize needs and potential problem areas during implementation and can save time and effort during implementation. The result is a more efficient and welcomed CR.

On-site education can be approached in many ways. An introduction to computers can be taught, preferably by the CR staff. The course should cover fundamentals of computer hardware, software, and user responsibilities and should describe the necessary interaction with the CR personnel. The material presented in the course should conform to the basic CR needs of those attending. For instance, physicians should learn the clinical uses of various CRs and the many methods for data input into and output from computer resources. Voice entry and reporting, light pen use, and passwords to restrict access and provide audit trails are but a few items of importance to this specific group of users. Physicians should be made aware of alternative methods for placing patient test requests into the computer and the current state of each method's technology. Often professional journals discuss unique and innovative ways to retrieve and view results when these methods may not be ready for everyday use. Physicians should also learn the limits of CRs. For example, prior visit patient test results may not be available because of limits to computer storage capacity.

Senior and middle managers should know their role in the selection, installation, and ongoing CR process. Staff persons must know their responsibility both during and after a CR is installed. Other topics may include what user methods will change under a computer system. Users should be concerned with what happens if there is a problem with the system's operation, such as when alternative backup methods are necessary when the computer is not functioning. The instructor should address the concerns and responsibility of each attendee while providing an overview of CR concepts and how they apply to the user and the organization.

An on-site education session is also an opportune time for one to make potential users aware of concerns that must be addressed before the installation of a CR. For instance, staffing and policy changes, facility needs, and other concerns can be freely discussed during classroom type presentations.

Figure 4-1 is a sample course agenda. Health-care case studies and literature should be used for discussion and to explain and demonstrate CR concepts.

Managers and supervisors with minimal experience with CR applications should be the first to attend the sessions. A seven-hour course offered in one-hour segments each week will provide a solid foundation for a team approach to the successful implementation of a CR. Persons attending the sessions can be given a Certificate of Achievement to demonstrate their learned computer literacy.

Literature that offers experiences with and methods for user applications and concerns can be distributed. For example, there are various approaches to selecting a laboratory system, and different laboratory vendors and packages have different capabilities. Exposing laboratory staff to various vendor approaches will make them more aware of the features and alternatives of different systems, a necessary prelude to the process of defining laboratory needs. Further, this begins the recognition of potential implementation problems that will need to be addressed in the installation planning process. The literature will also make the staff aware of the experiences of their peers and of the scope of interaction and user commitment necessary to ensure a successful (and even not so successful!) implementation and usage of the central CR staff.

Although there are staffing costs associated with users who are away from their jobs to attend classes, these are more than offset by the availabil-

Figure 4-1. Course agenda: Introduction to computers. Reprinted from *The Health Care Supervisor*, Volume 1, Number 4, July 1983, page 89, with permission of Aspen Publishers, Inc.

Class 1 Introduction
- Purpose of course
- Basic computer processes
  - Input
  - Output
  - Central Processing Unit (CPU)
    - Memory
    - Controller
    - Arithmetic/logic
- Manual versus computer processes
- Advantages of computerization
- Interaction
- DP vs CR vs DSS vs IS and other department titles

Class 2 Methods of Input and Output
- Disks
  - Fixed
  - Removable
  - Optical
- Microfiche
- Voice
- Magnetic tape
- Telecommunications
- OCR
- MCR
- Others
- Sample media and usage examples

Class 3 A Microcomputer Policy
- Why a policy
- The microcomputer policy
- Instituting the policy

Class 4 Computer Software
- What is software?
- Operating software
- Application software

Class 5 Types of Computer Installations
- Shared
- Service bureau
- Facilities management
- On-site
  - Centralized
  - Decentralized
  - Distributive
  - Turnkey
- UCRM and CCRM responsibilities

Figure 4-1, continued.

Class 6 Selecting a Computer Resource
- Interaction
- Identify needs
- Priorities
- RFP
- Proposal evaluations
- Selection

Class 7 The Computer Resource Life Cycle
- Inception
- Feasibility study
- System analysis
- System design
- System development
- Training, conversion, and installation
- Operations: the ongoing system
- Postimplementation analysis

ity of people who understand the value of computer resources and their role in its selection, installation, operation, and usage. In addition, when classes are presented by the CR staff, users and the CR staff will develop a rapport and confidence in each other. The users will see that the CR staff is concerned with the users' needs and is committed to user satisfaction. The bottom line of mutual cooperation is a workable and successful CR.

The Study Objective

In the development of a computer resource plan, the following process will identify short- and long-range information needs to support current and future plans and goals of both the organization and user. The method presented does not depend on whether an organization uses on-site or outside CR consultants. A properly planned CR can effectively assist in the delivery of patient care, affect user productivity, curtail and reduce costs, provide decision support data, and provide operational and managerial control. The planning study will also identify present and potential CR constraints such as timeframes, finances, user capabilities and commitment, staff and facility requirements.

The method also addresses changes to current manual and automated resources necessary for compatibility with future CR requirements. A systems plan will be prepared to show which applications and users should be automated, identify the costs and benefits associated with each application, and specify tentative implementation schedules.

When an organization chooses to use a consulting firm for all or part of a project, a key management person must be assigned to coordinate the project. This person is either the user computer resource manager (UCRM) or the central computer resource manager (CCRM) described in Chapter 2 with the appropriate qualifications and responsibilities.

The Role of the Steering Committee

The existence of a steering committee (as described in Chapter 2) is necessary in any process that will result in the selection and implementation of an organization-wide CR. When competition exists for limited computer resources and budgets, the committee will have the important task of assigning application priorities and selecting vendors. Furthermore, the committee members will be responsible for seeing that their respective areas participate effectively in the definition, implementation, and postinstallation phases.

The committee is composed of senior and middle managers. The steering committee should be able to give a proper hearing to all applications and vendors and assure that priority decisions are objective, politically acceptable, financially feasible, and appropriate to the organization's strategic business plan. The committee's assigned goals and responsibilities should be defined at the beginning of the project.

Because the CR study to be undertaken will have an impact on the entire organization, it must be carefully defined. Each user and application must be identified and prioritized as to its importance to the organization's strategic business plan. Committee members must therefore be capable of communicating within all levels of the organization and must be fully aware of overall organization objectives. The CCRM may serve as secretary of the committee and record meeting minutes.

Other members may include management personnel from nursing and ancillary services, the chief financial officer, and a member of the medical staff. The consultant, if retained, will be a member or advisor, as determined by the committee.

Other representatives can be called upon by the committee as necessary and may or may not become permanent members. As the project progresses into the later stages, usually past the priority phase, the committee may decide that line managers from the areas that will be directly affected by the project should become ad hoc members of the committee because the selection of vendors and applications will be essential to their areas and because their cooperation and esprit de corps will be required. However, the decision to include line managers must be made based on the capabilities of each individual line manager of each area. The CR project to be undertaken will require people capable of working together to achieve organization goals, not personal goals.

Some organizations may choose a committee that includes a trustee to provide liaison with the board of directors and to represent the board's goals and needs. A physician will do likewise for the medical staff. Each committee member must seek input from all levels of the organization for which he or she is responsible.

The committee must be educated to the potential and benefits of CR applications within the health-care environment. The committee should also be aware of the commitment, time, and funding necessary for successful computer resources. This knowledge can be obtained from literature on health-care CR applications and special instructional seminars. The CCRM should coordinate this progress. Suggested education methods are discussed earlier in this chapter.

Some people are mistakenly led to believe that one organization-wide CR is common throughout most organizations and further that these omnipresent applications are easily implemented and service all areas in an optimal manner. Through the technology of a database system, where all data are stored in one or many computers, an all-encompassing CR is, of course, theoretically possible. The literature frequently describes intensive systems that satisfy a variety of user needs, but the steering committee should be cautioned that these unique state-of-the-art systems are usually developed and installed over a period of years and are designed to fit the specific needs and management style of each organization. The implementation of these systems at other organizations is usually complex and requires extensive planning and effort. The introduction of microcomputer technology offers many users a degree of independence not available with centrally managed computers. All of these concerns and the accompanying benefits and problems—locally managed versus centrally managed—must be recognized by the committee.

Single vendors that offer multiple user applications usually recommend a modular approach with one or more databases serving as the foundation for all application modules, although one application is to be installed at a time. In this manner, the user and CR staff can serially become accustomed to the many new changes. This modular approach for an organization-wide CR will mean that the steering committee must prioritize and schedule applications to coincide and be consistent with the organization's long-range strategic plans and objectives. Thus, the CCRM may often need to educate the committee to help them understand the realities of real-world applications and provide a basis for determining time schedules and anticipating system complexities.

The sequence in which modular applications are scheduled must also be considered by the steering committee. For instance, a patient registration module should precede the radiology reporting module so that the registration system can provide patient identification data automatically to the radiology module.

The initial meeting of the steering committee should set the tone for the project, and it is essential that the CCRM and chairperson be well prepared for the meeting. They must understand the full scope of the project to be undertaken, as well as the CR manager's responsibility to the committee, and be ready to answer any questions raised by the committee, particularly regarding the availability, expertise, and cost of CR staff.

Several items should be on the agenda for the first meeting. First, the steering committee must understand the organization's current computer applications and staff resources. Second, the committee must clearly understand the goals and objectives of the study.

Third, the role that the committee will play in the project must be clearly discussed and defined so that the CR users and staff and the committee are aware of each other's responsibilities. The committee members must be aware that they are an integral part of the decision-making (or recommendation) process and that they are essential to assure that all personnel in the organization provide input to the planning process on a timely and accurate basis. For instance, the medical staff representative must survey his or her peers to make sure that the clinician's needs are addressed by the committee. The physician member of the committee must have the time to carry out this responsibility.

Each member of the steering committee should be made aware that demands for information will be made on both them and their subordinates to assure the preparation of a comprehensive systems plan. At this first meeting, the committee may be asked to identify key users to be interviewed regarding CR needs.

At subsequent meetings, the steering committee will review the CR staff findings regarding user information needs and CR applications, review user evaluations and application recommendations, and determine user application priorities and implementation schedules. The recommended processing approach to managing, controlling, and using the CRs (centralization and/or distribution of the computer resources, as will be discussed in Chapter 7) will be reviewed and approved by the committee.

Additional responsibilities of the committee will include conducting vendor interviews and evaluations, applying weighting factors to various application and vendor features, assessing vendor presentations, and, finally, selecting finalist vendors. The committee will also make site visits to finalist vendor installations. During the implementation of the CR, the steering committee will be responsible for monitoring schedule adherence and the successes (and failures!) of the system.

Determining Information Problems and Needs

Any organization considering the acquisition or upgrading of computer systems must identify the extent of services needed before it can decide whether these services can best be provided by an in-house staff or an outside computer service. Before these decisions, however, the organization must know the status of its present information systems—both automated and manual. This is accomplished with a systems study that defines and documents all current information procedures.

The study will identify present information system deficiencies and problems. This will guide the steering committee and the CR staff in later determining what additions and changes are necessary for future CR services. This method will also document and determine the scope of current CR services, the effectiveness of these services, and the CR staff's ability and resources to handle both current and future CR needs.

The study will also reveal users who are not ready to handle the responsibility of computerization. Some users have problems and needs beyond the scope of computerization. For these areas, management, operational policies, and procedures may need to be revamped before a computerized CR can be effective. For example, if a user area has excessive personnel turnover, a new information system has a high chance of failure because there is no lasting user continuity. The study may reveal that the high turnover probably has led to undocumented procedures and possibly a management that has not enforced compliance with new procedures or that is not capable of handling conflicts during implementation. If this area is to be selected for computerization, these internal problems must be solved first.

An example of where a study may identify system deficiencies that should be addressed before computerization is the manual billing system that produces incorrect patient bills. A study may indicate that the cause of the problem is the staff not submitting proper, chargeable procedures in a timely manner; thus, computerization will not eliminate these incomplete bills. The billing system should first be subject to an intensive systems study, and appropriate procedural changes should be made before computerization can be further considered.

If a laboratory has problems with equipment failure, computerization cannot solve the problem of incomplete and untimely patient test results caused by the laboratory equipment. The equipment problem must be repaired before a computer interface should be considered.

Any method used to identify and define organization-wide computer information needs must also be able to identify potential users for a CR application, as well as areas that need extensive study to correct operational deficiencies before computerization is considered. Further, many users may not be aware of how CR applications can be used or how their needs are common to other users. Thus, the approach to selecting CR applications should recognize each user's information problems and needs, regardless of whether those users seem to be candidates for computerization. Looking at organization-wide information needs in this manner will often reveal users with similar information problems and needs. Thus, what appears from individual user perspectives as a multitude of systems may in fact be one system that can satisfy the needs of many.

For example, the medical staff may request more timely patient radiology reports. In turn, the radiology department may have identified a need to enhance the method of preparing radiology reports. What first appeared as different uses and needs is now recognized as one common problem and need—timely radiology reporting.

The flow of data and information can be charted throughout the organization and used to identify common elements. The interview form (Figures 4-2 and 4-3) is one method that can be used to identify common data needs and problems among users. This may also reveal a user who was not initially considered to need access to a CR application. For example, in one hospital the volunteer department may need to access the real-time patient information system because it is responsible for distributing patient mail and a patient's in-house location is necessary information for this task. The public relations department may need to know in-house VIPs. The social service department may need information to screen for patients who are not currently receiving social service assistance, but who, because of certain criteria, should be. Initially, these three areas may not have been thought to have a need for CR services, but the needs definition study showed that they have needs similar to those of the laboratory—knowing a patient's location. Thus, identifying organization-wide information needs and then determining users can maximize the usage and justification of CR applications by making them available to all potential users.

Tracking information flow from data origin to usage areas may also uncover duplication of data sources, storage, and utilization. Tracking will also probably show that users with similar data needs usually have the same data problems: lack of accuracy or timeliness and an incompatibility with the other users' data sources. The flow analysis can later be used in preparation of a systems plan by identifying which areas can update the database and which users should only be able to access the data. For example, a hospital may determine that it is best to allow only the patient

Figure 4-2. Health-care CR interview guide instructions.

Interview Guide Instructions

Purpose: To determine:

- Your information needs.
- The method by which the needs are currently being met.
- The problems and possible improvements in meeting these needs

Present Information Needs:

List the primary information needs of your area. These are the items supplied to you from another area, put together in your area, and/or given by you to another area. They are the data that you must have to handle your assigned responsibility. You may do work on these needs, make decisions by them, or create work for another area. You may also list needs that are not currently being met. For example, a nurse station has a need to order laboratory tests, to provide patient conditions, to view patient demographic data, to update nursing notes, etc. A statistician uses various end-user workload statistics, comparative year-to-date data, occupancy statistics, etc. A physician's office needs date of last visit, diagnosis, prognosis, exams taken, etc.

THE REMAINING QUESTIONS ARE DIRECTED TO THE METHODS THAT ARE USED TO MEET EACH NEED.

Media that provide need? Log, report, telephone, etc.

List all logbooks, reports, documents, telephones,or other media that assist you in meeting the previously mentioned information need. There may be a number of ways used to meet one need.

THE REMAINING QUESTIONS ARE TO BE ANSWERED FOR EACH MEDIUM THAT YOU HAVE JUST LISTED.

Who uses medium? How is it used?

For each medium listed, state people who could use medium and how the medium is used in meeting the information need.

Who originates medium?

For each medium, state the user who prepares the medium and, if applicable, the area that receives the medium from you.

How is medium filed?

Do you keep the medium in alphabetical order, by state, by latest copy, etc.?

Frequency of update/usage/delivery?

How often do you receive each medium? How often is it used? Do you alter the medium in any way by additions, subtractions, or changes?

Figure 4-2, continued.

Do you use all data on the medium? If no, what?

Are you getting more information than you can use? Are you getting a report with a great deal of data and yet use only a small part of it?

Is this medium necessary? Is it timely and reliable?

Now that you have thought about the report, is it necessary? Is it getting to you on time so that the data are current for your needs? Are the data on the medium usually accurate? Can you depend on it?

Recommend improvements. How can the computer help?

This is your chance to give your thoughts on how your information needs can be improved by changing, adding, deleting, or combining this document, either manually or by other means. Can computers assist you? Do you know of a specific computer application?

---

registration department to make changes to a patient location, rather than allow multiple nursing units to handle this function as it would be difficult to pinpoint responsibility and accountability if census problems occurred. Nursing, however, may use the system for inquiry as to patient locations, while still being required to make all patient location change requests through the patient registration department. The information flow analysis can also be used when determining a user's hardware needs, such as visual display terminals (VDTs), printers, and microcomputers.

Identifying organization-wide CR needs and problems requires that key personnel from each user area identify their current information needs and their problems in meeting them. These personnel can be line management, members of the medical staff, and other appropriate personnel knowledgeable about how an area functions. The people to be interviewed do not need to have an understanding of computer applications, but must know their area's operations and current information needs.

The interview form to identify information needs is one method of collecting data that will identify common user information problems and needs. Getting people to discuss all of the ideas and needs they handle routinely is often difficult, and the interview form must be designed so that it follows as closely as possible the logical thought process of information usage. The form should request a list of all reports used or created within the area of responsibility, regardless of whether the interviewee thinks that the need can be computerized. The form should request the area and method that supplies the information and ask the user to identify any problems with

Present Information Need	Media That Provide Need? Log, Rpt, Tel., Etc.	Who Uses Media? How Used?	Who Originates Media?	How Are Media Filed?	Do You Use All Data on Media? If No, What?	Frequency of Update,Use, Delivery?	Are These Media Necessary, Timely & Reliable?	Please Recommend Improvements. Can the Computer Help?

Name ______________ Area Representing ______________

Figure 4-3. Computer Resource Interview Guide.

using the information. A problem that makes the information questionable or not usable should be explained. Problems can generally be categorized (accuracy, timeliness, completeness, etc.).

A nurse may identify an information need, i.e., requesting from the laboratory a patient blood test. This information need may be met through a request slip prepared by the nurse and sent through transport services or hand-carried, or the request may be telephoned. A problem with this method may be a delay in getting the request to the laboratory. The test can also be delayed by the laboratory because the patient data supplied by the nurse is incomplete, perhaps lacking the patient's weight and height. These problems should be listed on the form with the identified need.

In a large organization, 25 to 40 people may be interviewed, necessitating group presentations. At other times the form may be explained to users in individual sessions. The form should have written instructions and examples. The examples should be further discussed at the meetings. Each person should have at least a week to complete the form, after which staff will meet with the person a second time to obtain an explanation and an understanding of each area's information requirements and problems.

In the second meeting, the analyst will summarize for each user the problems described. At a third meeting, the analyst will present written documentation of how the CR staff perceived the user's problems, as well as the CR staff's proposed automation recommendations to the user (Figure 4-4). This summary discussion will usually result in changes to the problems and automation needs. Essentially, the summary is the CR staff's understanding of the end-user's information needs and problems. It offers the user an opportunity to discuss how computers can be used in the area and lets the CR staff react to these ideas from the central planning perspective. This approach educates the users and starts them thinking about how automation can assist them in meeting information needs, while also allowing the CR staff to discuss integrated and other user's potential automation needs with the user. This technique is simply one of using CR and user staff interaction to begin the process of identifying unique CR applications for computerization.

This approach will also identify information problems and needs that can be solved immediately, without waiting for computerization. For example, nursing may identify a daily statistical report as being inaccurate and never used. The staff might determine that the report is inaccurate because of obsolete calculations and might take action immediately to use updated formulas. Other reports may be identified as untimely, and the solution may be simply to change a scheduled delivery time. Sometimes needs believed not available by one user, such as a report on employee vacation and sick hours, may be readily available to another user, and the solution may be to prepare an extra copy for distribution.

Figure 4-4. Perceived problems of same day surgical (SDS) registration in fiscal year 1990 (key volumes: 1,009 same day surgical admissions) and proposed automation needs.

OPERATING PROBLEMS:

1. Maintaining timely census of full and empty beds and location of patients; notifying of discharges, transfers, and pending discharges
2. Getting medical record to patient area as soon as possible
3. Registering patient quickly with accurate data; getting patient information (DOB, religion, previous admission, etc.)
4. Holding prior SDS test results until patient arrives; having incomplete results when patient arrives
5. Initiating the ordering of tests
6. Having patient condition information available to assist in discharging
7. Making identification plate for each patient

PERCEIVED AUTOMATED NEEDS:

1. When patient gives name and DOB or patient provides Medical identification card, system will recall demographic information for registration. As clerk enters additional or new data, system will edit data for completeness and accuracy. Patient will automatically be entered in census and financial systems.
2. Tests for surgical admissions will be generated.
3. Nurse will screen via computer preadmission SDS results for incomplete and positive test results before patient arrives.
4. Census will be kept on computer, and computer will note appropriate patient location.
5. Medical records will automatically be notified of emergency for record retrieval.
6. Computer will hold 3SU and preadmission patient information until patient is admitted.
7. Access to OR schedule for information will be possible.
8. Access to physicians who are on-call or in-house will be possible.
9. Statistics (type of operative procedure, visits by service, etc.) will be available.
10. Physicians can access patient demographics and tests via computer directly from their offices.

The final summary report of the perceived problems and proposed automation needs should be returned to the user for signed approval. The user should be instructed to return the approved summary within a set time, usually a week. This written response is the user's commitment that the user's information needs and problems have been identified, understood by the analyst, and discussed with the user.

In summary, identifying the information needs and problems of an organization involves four steps:

Step 1. The CR staff explains the purpose of the study and form. Each user area has at least a week to complete the problems and needs form.

Step 2. The CR staff meets with each user a second time to discuss the user's information needs and problems.

Step 3. At a third meeting, the CR staff presents its perceived problems and proposed automation needs for discussion and approval.

Step 4. The list of perceived problems and proposed automation needs is given written approval by the user.

It is important that these steps not be rushed. The four steps can take four to six weeks per user area. Interaction is now working.

Identifying Automation Needs

The report of perceived problems and automation needs can be reviewed with members of the CR staff, the consultant, the user, and/or the steering committee to identify and categorize the common information needs and problems. This process will result in the definition of many unique CR needs such as patient registration and scheduling, laboratory test reporting, payroll/personnel overtime usage, pharmacy drug formulary, order entry, case mix analysis, etc. One means to accomplish this process of CR application definition is the matrix shown in Figure 4-5, which can be prepared using each needs report as input. As each report's needs and problems are discussed, they can be classified into unique applications. This review process continues as each report and each user's need and problem is compared with the matrix. If the matrix does not already list the user's need, then another information application has been identified.

Identifying the Type and Maturity of User Computer Applications

When discussing whether a user should consider computerization, one needs to know the available applications and the features that they commonly provide. One needs to know the user applications that are in the conception stage (the very beginning stage of development) and that may not be practical for consideration at this time. For example, on-line registration is a computer application considered to be matured. It is widely

USER AREA	VDTs	PRINTERs	COMPUTER APPLICATIONS Inpatient registration	Outpatient registration	Order entry & results reporting	Pharmacy	Laboratory
Registration	18	4	X	X	X		
Pharmacy	10	5	X	X	X	X	X
Medical records	4	2	X	X	X	X	X
Laboratory	34	10	X	X	X	X	X
Information desk	2	1	X	X			
Utilization review	3	1	X	X	X	X	X

During the review of each user's perceived problems and proposed automated solution list, the above matrix worksheet is updated and continually revised. For example, a registration application will provide certain functions (i.e., collects patient demographic data and maintains patient location). An X is placed under the COMPUTER APPLICATIONS column across from Pharmacy to show that this user area will have a need to access this application.

The numbers listed under VDT and PRINTER are the estimates of how many of these units will be needed in the user area.

Figure 4-5. User area needs as a function of computer applications.

available in many different health organizations and is offered by a multitude of software vendors. Among its features are retrieval of previously collected patient demographic data and a capability of interfacing with other mature applications, such as patient billing. On the other hand, an application such as computer storage and retrieval of roentgenograms is still being developed and is offered by only a limited number of vendors.

Published surveys (Packer 1988; Dorenfest et al. 1987) provide a perspective as to commonly available applications. Users can evaluate their staff's level of computer maturity and then decide whether it is practical to consider automation. Computer-assisted literature searches can be a valuable resource for a user evaluating the maturity and scope of a specific application. Examples of search criteria are computers and hospitals, computers and nursing homes, computers and home visits, and computers and HMOs. A general search can show the extent of computerization in a particular health-care industry, and then one can refine the search to specific end-user applications. A literature search in conjunction with surveys showing numbers of users of the application provides a reference for users to determine whether they wish to proceed slowly or immediately with automation.

With this method what may initially have appeared as, for example, 25 user areas with 25 unique needs and problems, gradually becomes recognizable as many common items shared throughout the organization. The 25 users interviewed may have common needs that can be satisfied with the five functions listed in the matrix of Figure 4-5. The repetitive documentation for this process is a necessary step. It will put into perspective for the CR staff and steering committee the users who can utilize computerized CR services and will also help in determining application priorities and implementation schedules.

The final matrix can now be presented to the steering committee to show the scope of users interviewed and the common need of many of the users for the same information. This matrix presents a picture of how the various CR applications can relate to the total organization. It will now be the committee's responsibility to rank the identified applications.

Prioritizing Automation Needs

The purpose of prioritization is to rate each application as to its ability to meet the organization's strategic business plan. Each application, or module, should be examined for its effect on management decision-making, time necessary for implementation, improvement in quality of patient care/satisfaction, enhancement of public relations, effect on employee morale, and financial impact on present and future revenues and costs. Installing all applications simultaneously is usually impractical and thus the prioritization and scheduling of each application individually is required.

One method for evaluating multiple CR applications and comparing them against each other is to evaluate each application using economic and patient care index factors (Figure 4-6). This method allows committee members to rank each application according to perceived effect on the organization economically and in quality of care.

The ranking procedure is designed to provide a methodical and forced approach to ranking a multitude of applications. For instance, a person asked to prioritize 14 applications from one through 14 will often find the task time-consuming and the end results rather arbitrary. The recommended method forces the ranker to consider each application on its own merit, which in this example gives us two perspectives—economic and patient care (Figures 4-6 and 4-7). Other perspectives (such as employee and patient morale) can be included if desired.

The composite score for all members' rankings (Figure 4-8) is presented at a committee meeting for discussion, modification, and final committee approval. The committee's discussion of the final ranking should focus on demonstrable computer system costs of each system, space constraints in the organization, time needed to implement the system, difficulty of implementation, an end-user's ability to provide interaction, and even political considerations. It may also be decided to postpone making a decision to acquire the lower ranked applications. However, the lower ranked applications can be included in the CR long-range plan, as is discussed in Chapter 8. This will allow the applications acquired today to interface with the expected CR needs of the future.

It is at this stage of the project, after the applications have been prioritized, that the committee may want to expand its membership to include line managers who will be utilizing the potential new applications. On the other hand, these line managers could simply be included as guests at all meetings. In either case, rather than have the committee force a computer vendor or application on a user, the user should be given ample opportunity to provide input to the committee as well as to acquire an in-depth understanding of the priorities and selection criteria used by the committee.

Figure 4-6. Memo to the steering committee giving instructions on how to rank system functions.

SYSTEM FUNCTION RANKING PROCEDURE

TO: Steering Committee Members

FROM:

SUBJECT: System function Rankings

The purpose of this memo is to explain the method that should be used to rank each of the major system functions. This, in turn, will identify the organization's system plan and provide input for assessing the cost of various alternatives.

In developing your rankings, the following steps should be used:

STEP 1. Read the systems synopsis of each system function. This will familiarize each member with the benefits of the function and what the automated system is intended to do.

STEP 2: Assign an economic value to each system function and record in the column on Worksheet 1 entitled "Economic Value Index." Economic values used should correspond to the following list based upon your opinion as to the economic value of the system to the organization. Vales to be used are:

= 3 if system function has *high* economic value
= 2 if system function has *moderate* value
= 1 if system function has *low* value
= 0 if system function has *very low* value

STEP 3. Assign a quality of care patient satisfaction index value to each function. The following values should be used and placed in the column entitled "Quality of Care/ Satisfaction Index."

= 3 if system function will *greatly increase* the qualify of care being given or patient satisfaction
= 2 if system function will *moderately increase* the quality of care being given or patient satisfaction
= 1 if system function will *slightly increase* care or patient satisfaction
= 0 if system function will *maintain the level* of care/patient satisfaction or will not increase care quality/satisfaction whatsoever.

STEP 4. Add the Economic Index and Quality of Care/Satisfaction Index together and record the answer in the column headed "Total Index."

STEP 5. From Worksheet #1, select the functions with the highest total index (i.e. those that = 6) and list those functions' letter designations under the column headed "Priority Level #1" on Worksheet #2.

Select the functions with the next highest total index (i.e., those that = 5) and list their letter designations under "Priority Level #2."

Select the remaining functions under (=3, =2, =1) and list under "Priority Level #3."

STEP 6. Using Worksheet #2, within each priority level, numerically rank each function in order of importance to the organization in your opinion. In other words, all functions under Priority Level #1 equaling 6 should be ranked in importance to the organization.

Each level has been determined to have a meaning to the organization and all functions in that group will take on that significance in the final systems plan.

Figure 4-6, continued.

STEP 7. On Worksheet #1, fill in the Final Rank column as determined from Worksheet #2.

You have now ranked all of major system functions for the organization, and your rankings will provide input to a composite ranking to be reviewed with the committee.

Thank you.

Figure 4-7. Worksheets #1 and #2 for systems function ranking. Reprinted with permission of A. T. Kearney, Inc.

Systems Function Ranking Worksheet #1

Major Systems Functions	Economic Value Index	Quality of Care/Satisfaction Index	Total Index	Final Rank
A. Census and Bed	____	____	____	____
B. Patient Registration & Data Collection	____	____	____	____
C. Patient Scheduling	____	____	____	____
D. Order Entry/Charge Collection	____	____	____	____
E. Operating Statistics	____	____	____	____
F. Laboratory	____	____	____	____
G. Radiology Reporting	____	____	____	____
H. Medical Data Collection and Record Retrieval	____	____	____	____
I. Pharmacy	____	____	____	____
J. MD Location/Messages	____	____	____	____
K. Inventory	____	____	____	____
L. Engineering Maintenance	____	____	____	____
M. Employee Staffing and Scheduling	____	____	____	____
N. Employee Stats/Info	____	____	____	____

Systems Function Ranking Worksheet #2

PRIORITY LEVEL #1		PRIORITY LEVEL #2		PRIORITY LEVEL #3	
Total Index = 6		Total Index = 4–5		Total Index = 1–3	
Function Letter	Numerical Rank	Function Letter	Numerical Rank	Function Letter	Numerical Rank
____	____	____	____	____	____
____	____	____	____	____	____

Figure 4-8. Computer resource priorities ranking summary.

	Rater								Composite		Consultant		Total	
	1	2	3	4	5	6	7	8	Index	Rank	Index	Rank	Index	Rank
A. Census and bed control	1	7	4	2	5	1	1	6	5.0	4				
B. Patient registration data collection	4	4	6	3	3	2	6	1	5.25	1				
C. Patient scheduling	8	3	10	9	7	9	8	2	4.37	7				
D. Order entry/charge collection	2	5	7	1	6	3	2	3	5.12	2				
E. Operating statistics	9	10	13	13	13	9	12	4	2.75	11				
F. Laboratory	5	1	2	6	1	4	4	11	5.12	3				
G. Radiology reporting	6	8	8	4	12	7	7	12	4.0	8				
H. Medical data collection and medical record retrieval	3	2	11	5	11	5	5	8	4.62	6				
I. Pharmacy	7	6	3	8	2	6	3	9	4.87	5				
J. MD location/messages	13	11	14	14	14	11	14	7	1.75	14				
K. Inventory	10	9	5	12	8	12	13	10	3.12	10				
L. Engineering/maintenance	14	12	12	11	9	14	10	14	2.12	13				
M. Employee staffing and scheduling	11	13	1	7	4	10	11	5	4.0	9				
N. Employee stats/info	12	14	9	10	10	13	9	13	2.37	12				

The Systems Plan

Once the steering committee prioritizes the CR applications and requirements, the CR staff can proceed to determine the most feasible generic processing alternative (such as outside service, in-house, facilities management, networked microcomputers, mainframe computer, distributed minicomputers, upgrade or maintain existing hardware). Hardware, software, and personnel costs for each alternative must be estimated, and implementation timeframes must be determined. The alternatives must be presented to the steering committee, and the CR staff must be prepared to recommend one or two of the alternatives. The committee must determine its priorities relative to cost and implementation timeframes. (See Chapters 6 and 7 for more detailed presentations on the computer system life cycle and the centralization and distribution of CR resources.)

The completed systems plan will be a comprehensive, practical system development effort that details future CR development, installation tasks, and tentative timetables. The systems plan may now need to be presented to the Chief Executive Officer and/or the Board of Trustees for approval. Further, the plan, depending on its costs, may need the approval of state and/or federal agencies. If this is the case, it will probably need refinements to conform to their reporting requirements.

Although explained briefly here, the development of the comprehensive systems plan is tedious and time-consuming. Evaluation of generic alternatives and presentation to the committee can require two to four months of extensive systems analysis, depending on the CR staff and experience. Texts are available for further detail of this method.

Request for Proposal

Once the steering committee, chief executive officer, and/or board has approved the systems plan, the organization can begin to solicit vendor proposals for hardware and software. This process is usually accomplished with a request for proposal (RFP). A RFP explains in explicit terms to a potential vendor the organization's strategic business plan, CR needs, systems plan, and priorities. In addition, the RFP provides guidelines for the organization to measure a vendor's ability to provide the required CR functions. Many times a vendor's willingness to comply with the RFP format itself is an indication of the future vendor/organization relationship.

Minicase 2: Absence and Presence of a Request for Proposal

Explaining to a vendor the information needs for a physician group practice CR and obtaining a verbal and inappropriately written response that does not address the group's needs can be a very frustrating experience. An example is a group practice that selected a computer application without the benefit of a RFP and the difficulty that resulted when the practice selected one vendor from several.

The group's manager interviewed five vendors and explained the group's CR needs and constraints. Each vendor supplied literature on its system's capability and responded that the system could meet all of the group's information needs. In addition, the vendor's responses went into detail not pertinent to the group's needs. After each interview, the manager was certain that the last vendor was the best one, but it was never clear that the vendor really understood the group's CR needs. The manager had a sense that the facility and staff limits were not clear to the vendor.

The group was in a turmoil trying to decide which vendor could best meet its CR needs. To eliminate this frustration, the group manager decided to prepare a brief, almost apologetic, RFP outlining the required applications needs. Each vendor was asked to respond to the RFP. The manager used this method to quantify the vendor responses so that each vendor's capabilities could be compared with the required needs. The verbal responses and digressions from the specific needs still made it difficult to identify the vendor able to satisfy the group's needs.

Finally, a detailed RFP was prepared and vendors were required to respond in writing and in a fixed format. The group manager was now able to compare the five vendors equally to determine their ability to meet the cost and needs constraints. This method resulted in two of the five vendors meeting the requirements. Of these two vendors, one's cost was significantly lower than the other while the ability to meet other requirements (such as delivery time, service, education training, etc.) was equal for both vendors. The physician group was now able to feel confident in the selection of a vendor that could satisfy its needs at a reasonable cost.

RFP Preparation

When preparing a RFP, there are many possible formats. One recommended method is to review the formats of RFPs that similar size organizations have used in order to ensure that all areas of concern are addressed in the RFP. Vendors frequently respond only to questions asked, and the organization may not be aware of other concerns until it faces an unforeseen expense or problem. There is a need to present RFP questions clearly and specifically. Reviewing RFPs that have been prepared by other organizations before preparing one's own RFP can ensure that all areas of concern are addressed.

A RFP can be prepared by the CR and user staff or by the consultant and be approved by the steering committee. Figure 4-9 shows a sample table of contents for a RFP.

A letter of transmittal can accompany the RFP to invite potential vendors to submit proposals. The letter should note the date when the vendors' proposals are needed and to whom the proposals should be addressed. Other appropriate schedule dates, such as when equipment and applications are needed, can be listed. Both the letter and the RFP should state that all proposals submitted become the property of the organization. The letter should specify the one person who will answer all vendor questions. Usually this person is the CCRM. This prevents vendors from making numerous calls to users, trustees, and senior management in an attempt to influence these members. The letter should also emphasize that the written proposal must be in a specified format.

The introduction section of the RFP should explain the scope of the proposal and such items as time constraints and vendor evaluation criteria. It should summarize the required response formats of the proposed equipment/software/services. A timetable for proposal submissions, vendor meetings, and contract negotiations should be detailed. A table of contents should be available for easy vendor reference.

In the background section, the organization should be described in terms of its relationship to the community, services offered, number of employees, and other information necessary for the vendor to understand the strategic business plan, goals, and objectives of the organization. The organization's future CR plans should also be described. Sometimes it is helpful if the organization describes the factors that will shape the selection of a vendor, for example, 40% production functional capabilities, 15% implementation plan and disruption to user operation, etc.

A section should be included to explain appropriate volume and workload statistics such as patient days, clients seen, services performed, clinic visits, patients seen by each physician, employees, laboratory tests, etc. If there is an expected increase in services, it should be noted.

The history of computer resources at the organization should be explained, and current applications, hardware, and staff should be described. Hardware, software, and personnel costs should be detailed.

The systems plan section should discuss the plan as approved by the committee. It should explain the timing relationships, processing approach (such as distributed, centralized, shared, or outside vendor), and generally summarize the required application needs.

Figure 4-9. Table of Contents of a sample RFP. Reprinted from *Managing Hospital Information Systems* by S. L. Priest, p. 51. with permission of Aspen Publishers, Inc.

RFP
TABLE OF CONTENTS

The vendor proposal requirements section of the RFP should detail the required vendor written response formats. Figures 4-10 through 4-15 show sample vendor response formats for equipment prices, software prices, operating costs and charges, equipment and operating system descriptions, and physical plant requirements. This section will reveal the vendor's ability to meet the organization's needs. The responses must be in a format that allows the organization to compare the capabilities and costs of all vendors. The organization should not have to interpret vendor responses in order to compare capabilities and costs. For example, if vendor A responded with the total purchase price of the system and vendor B gave annual rental cost, the organization would have to interpret these costs to compare one to the other. If vendor A responded with separate maintenance costs and vendor B did not quantify maintenance costs, but included them with the system cost, it may appear that vendor B has higher system costs. Requiring all vendors to respond in the same format eliminates interpretation and prejudice by the person doing the analysis.

The vendor must be required to identify all costs that the organization could incur even if not specifically requested in the RFP. These include hardware, software, staffing, operating, maintenance, training, and any other possible costs. The RFP may even specify that costs not submitted by the vendor will be assumed to be included as part of the vendor's other costs.

The response formats must have the vendor respond to each output and input requirement in a manner that allows the organization to judge quickly the degree to which a vendor can meet a need. Within the RFP, however, the vendor should be able to supply additional information on the system's capabilities. Thus, the vendor is not restricted from recommending other approaches and needs that can further enhance the system, but the organization must determine where in the RFP these features are presented.

The vendor must explain its proposed hardware and software warranty performance, such as response time to software and hardware problems, and its proposal should include a copy of its standard contract. The RFP should note that both the vendor proposal and the RFP may become part of the final contract. Some vendors will take exception to having their standard contract altered, but inclusion of this statement in the RFP makes the vendor aware that you want responses backed up and supported by proven systems.

The vendor should supply the names of all existing clients, not just a selected number. It is also important that the vendor respond to system specifications only when the feature can be demonstrated. Responses of soon-to-be-released products may put the organization in a situation where it is testing the vendor's new products. Being a pilot site is justifiable under certain conditions, but the organization must be aware of the problems and confusion that accompany a test system.

Figure 4-10. Proposed equipment cost per year of a 5-year lease. Reprinted with permission of A. T. Kearney, Inc.

Item	First Year			Second Year			Third Year			Fourth Year			Fifth Year			Five-Year Total Cost
	No.	Unit Cost	Total Cost/ Year	No.	Unit Cost	Total Cost/ Year	No.	Unit Cost	Total Cost/ Year	No.	Unit Cost	Total Cost/ Year	No.	Unit Cost	Total Cost/ Year	
<u>Processing Unit(s)</u>																
<u>Storage Devices</u>																
Disk																
Tape																
Other (Specify)																
<u>Input/Output Devices</u>																
Key/Tape/Disk/Voice																
Other Reader																
Terminals																
VDT																
Printer																
Other (Specify)																
<u>Other (Specify)</u>																
<u>Additional Charges</u>																
Taxes																
Overtime Rental																
Freight																
Maintenance																
Other (Specify)																
Total																

Figure 4-11. Proposed software cost per year of a 5-year contract. Reprinted with permission of A. T. Kearney, Inc.

Item	First Year		Second Year		Third Year		Fourth Year		Fifth Year		
	Basic Unit Cost	Total Cost/ Year	Basic Unit Cost	Total Cost/ Year	Basic Unit Cost	Total Cost/ Year	Basic Unit Cost	Total Cost/ Year	Basic Unit Cost	Total Cost/ Year	Five-Year Total Cost
Operating Software (Specify Application)											
Inpatient Admitting											
Outpatient Registration/Scheduling											
Order Entry/Charge Collection											
Pharmacy											
Laboratory Reporting											
Additional Costs											
Report/Feature Options Not Reflected Above											
Taxes											
Extra Reports and Screening											
Other (Specify)											
Total											

Figure 4-12. Estimated annual operating costs and charges, 5-year plan. Reprinted with permission of A. T. Kearney, Inc.

Item	First Year			Second Year			Third Year			Fourth Year			Fifth Year			
	No.	Unit Cost	Total Cost/ Year	No.	Unit Cost	Total Cost/ Year	No.	Unit Cost	Total Cost/ Year	No.	Unit Cost	Total Cost/ Year	No.	Unit Cost	Total Cost/ Year	Five-Year Total Cost
Training (Vendor-provided)																
Nonchargeable Days/Year																
Chargeable Days/Year																
Installation and Support Assistance (Vendor-provided)																
Nonchargeable Days/Year																
Chargeable Days/Year																
Personnel (Facility or Vendor-provided)																
Management																
Programmer																
Systems Analyst																
Operator																
Clerical																
Other (Specify)																

Figure 4-13. Proposed equipment and operating system descriptions. Reprinted with permission of A. T. Kearney, Inc.

Item	Description/Operating Factors
Central (or Mini) Processing Units with Main Memory (speed, memory size)	
Storage Devices (size, access rate, medium file organization)	
Input/Output Devices (speed, medium, number required)	
Other (Specify)	
Operating Software Systems (for each application)	
Main Memory Size Requirements Language	
How Many Programs Can Be Operated Simultaneously?	
How Much Memory Available for Applications Programs?	
Can System Simultaneously Process Programs in Different Languages?	
Can System Segment Program To Process Larger than Available Memory Size Programs?	
Is System Upward-compatible?	
Is There a Memory Protect Feature?	

Figure 4-14. Estimated annual physical plant requirements. Reprinted with permission of A. T. Kearney, Inc.

Item	First Year	Second Year	Third Year	Fourth Year	Fifth Year
Square Feet					
Structure Requirements					
Utilities Equipment					
Uninterrupted Power Supply (UPS)					
A/C					
Electrical					
Other (Specify)					
Estimated Annual Depreciation Costs					

Figure 4-15. Vendor applications/systems presently available. Reprinted with permission of A. T. Kearney, Inc.

Application/System	Available? Yes	No	Comments or Description
1.0 Inpatient Admitting (indicate interface with financial systems)			
1.1 Preadmission Report (a)			
1.2 Bed Availability Report (a)			
1.3 Admission/Discharge/Transfer Report (a)			
1.4 Changed Admission Information Report (a)			

Code: (a) absolute; (h) highly desirable; (d) desirable.

Organizations desiring to contract with only one vendor may specify in the RFP that they will deal only with one primary vendor, although the vendor's proposed CR may be made up of other vendors' hardware and software. This minimizes the problems that can occur when an organization has to coordinate multivendors and the frustration of having to rectify the situation when one vendor feels that the other's product is causing a problem.

Training programs on site and at the vendor site should be explained along with additional costs. The response formats may even specify an equipment backup site to handle processing if there are long-term hardware problems. The equipment and software capabilities must include an ability to be upgraded. A CR application that is to be interfaced with additional or later applications, equipment, or databases must be demonstrable today.

The vendor's recommended implementation schedule should be included with the proposal and should detail both vendor and organization implementation and time limit responsibilities. In many cases, this will only be a representative schedule because there are so many variables, such as staff vacations, hardware delivery, vendor commitment to other contracts, etc. The organization should have final approval over all time schedules.

If the organization will need remedial maintenance during certain hours differing from the vendor's prime hours, the cost and availability of this service should be explained.

The total data processing section of the RFP must specify exactly what the organization expects each application to do. Figure 4-16 is a sample of a detail specification sheet for one input-output need. This layout details each output and input requirement. The vendor will explain its ability to meet each need. Each output requirement must have its degree of importance to the organization.

One may clarify the specifications and needs required of a CR application by sometime during the preparation of the RFP, asking the potential vendors to give presentations to the steering committee and other key personnel. The committee can then provide greater input during the needs definition stage of the RFP by being aware of available features versus features that are nondemonstrable today. This provides further insight into the types of CR that the organization may want to solicit from vendors.

The RFP usually does not detail hardware capabilities such as memory or disc capacities. These functions are determined by the vendor from the organization's computer resource priorities and needs. However, the RFP may specify the type of equipment, the operating system used, and in which language the application is programmed. This requirement depends on the organization's current hardware and software experience and capabilities.

The RFP should require that the vendor's proposed software and hardware demonstrate a minimal capability to process the organization's current input, storage, and access workloads. Further, the vendor should state its ability to handle additional workloads. This can be expressed in terms of percentages, such as "can handle a 45% increase in laboratory tests with proposed system."

The RFP may ask for resumes of vendor personnel who will be assigned to implement the system. With such information, one can determine their scope of experience and ability to communicate with organizational personnel. The organization may even want to interview vendor analysts to determine their ability to understand health-care terminology and process. Analysts should be experienced in the vendor's recommended hardware and software. Sometimes an inexperienced analyst acquires experience while the organization receives unplanned costs and frustrations and even ineffective systems.

Part of the time schedule in the RFP should include an initial vendor meeting. This meeting, as explained in the transmittal letter, is to answer the questions of vendors who are interested in responding to the RFP. The

Figure 4-16. Systems input/output specifications. Reprinted with permission of A. T. Kearney, Inc.

BASIC APPLICATION: Inpatient Admitting **FEATURE TITLE:** Admission/Discharge/ Transfer Inquiry

PURPOSE: Provide information on patient census status (A,D,T)
Requesting prior medical records as appropriate
Have data-edit capabilities

USAGE:		**DEGREE OF NEED:**		**DISTRIBUTION/ACCESS:**	
Plan	___	Absolute	X	Admitting	Info. Desk
Control	X	Highly Desirable	___	Patient Accounts	Housekeeping
Operational	X	Desirable	___	Medical Records	Volunteer Ofc.
				Physician	Pharmacy
				Dietary	Public Rel.
				Nursing	

FREQUENCY:				**DATA SEQUENCE OPTIONS:**
Daily	___	Quarterly	___	1. Patient name
Weekly	___	Annually	___	2. Patient number
Monthly	___	Request	X	3. Physician/patient name
		Other	___	4. Religion/patient name

Major Input Requirements: Item/Source	Number of Active Records	Number of Characters/Record	Present Storage Medium
Admission registration data	45	500	Disk Soundex System

MAJOR OUTPUT FIELD DESCRIPTIONS:

Patient biographical and demographic data
Service
Physician
Patient medical record/account number
Admission/discharge date-time
Room-bed assignment
Guarantor/insurance/employment information
Detail deposit and previous balance information
Admitting diagnosis/symptoms
Admission protocol
Patient financial classification data (9 categories)
Length of stay
From–to date on transfers
Control totals
Patient type
Stoppage of standard service orders upon discharge
Diagnosis
Pending discharge notification
Financial discharge clearance
Religion

meeting is to clarify problems with the RFP and to summarize areas of particular concern to the organization. Vendors may also be given a tour of the facility, and appointments can be set up for them to gather further information if necessary. The RFP should be reviewed and approved by the steering committee and potential users before being sent out.

Identifying Potential Vendors

Professional journals and texts can provide a wealth of information on vendors to which you may want to send a request for proposal (Higgins and Wilcox 1989; Dorenfest et al. 1987; Sneider 1987; Rowland and Rowland 1985). Published surveys of computer hardware and software vendors will provide data on degree of user satisfaction with a vendor's support and application features. Survey results often show whether a vendor's client base is increasing or decreasing, a fact important in determining the vendor clients' level of satisfaction with the vendor's ability to maintain a quality, state-of-the-art product.

One's auditing firm can usually provide a list of potential CR vendors. Professional associations, such as state associations and user groups, are an excellent source of potential vendors from whom to request a proposal. Conversation with users of a vendor's services will provide insights that can also be used in the final vendor selection process.

Conclusion

In this chapter, a sample methodology to identify an organization's computer resource priorities has been discussed. These priorities become part of the systems plan. A request for proposal (RFP) that details the priorities and the systems plan is prepared.

Frequently, an organization will select computer hardware and software first—before their actual needs are identified. This method can result in the computer not meeting the organization's present and future strategic business and CR plans, if indeed plans exist. The approach presented in this chapter stresses the importance of first defining existing and future information needs and problems. Only after the organization has identified its CR needs should software be selected. The hardware selection can be recommended by the vendor.

A consultant may be able to provide the organization with the experience and method necessary to identify and define the organization's CR needs and systems plan. The method explained in this chapter will generally apply whether the study is accomplished by in-house CR staff or with a consultant. The selection of a consulting firm should be made carefully and be dependent on fellow health facility references, cost, and previous experience in health-care CR needs.

In preparation for new and additional CR applications, the organization should encourage educational programs for potential users to understand basic CRs and computer concepts. This should include seminars on computers and on user and CR staff responsibilities and interaction. Appropriate literature on CR applications and problems should be reviewed and discussed.

The objective of a study to determine CR needs must be thoroughly understood by key organization personnel, particularly by senior management, the users involved, and the steering committee. CR needs should always coincide with the organization's short- and long-range strategic business plans. Each user must have a role in defining the information needs. A systems plan must be approved by the steering committee. This plan details the approach to and timeframe in implementing the committee's information recommendations.

The committee must review each phase of the project and participate in the needs definition and systems ranking function. To assist the committee in ranking priorities, a suggested method considers the potential CR effect on the organization's financial resources and patient care.

A system study puts into perspective the total effect of the CRs on the organization. This includes user procedure changes and staffing. It identifies areas that have to be corrected before computerization can occur and other potential problem areas. The study may identify economic and technological constraints that may limit the extent and complexity of a CR within the organization.

The request for proposal (RFP) presents the facilities' systems plan and CR priorities and specifies formats in which the vendor must respond. A required response format minimizes interpretation by the analyst of the vendor's responses regarding its ability to meet the RFP specifications and allows equitable evaluation and comparison of multiple vendors. The hardware and software to accomplish the required needs can frequently be chosen by the vendor. With this system, a vendor has more flexibility in proposing a CR system to meet the organization's needs. A vendor responding to a request for quote must choose from a narrower set of possibilities in molding a proposed solution.

Chapter 5 discusses an evaluation method that can be applied to selecting vendor proposals that have been sent to the organization in response to the organization's request for proposal.

Questions and Assignments

1. Break the class into groups of five to seven students. Assign each student a management position on a computer steering committee, i.e., chief financial officer, chief operating officer, central computer resource manager, vice president nursing, vice president clinical departments, trustee, chief of medicine, purchasing agent. Hand out a summary of the benefits and functions of six computer applications, i.e., laboratory, registration, radiology, accounting, pharmacy, and medical records. Hand out copies of the forms shown in Figures 4-6 to 4-8 and have members of the committee prioritize the applications as perceived by their new identities. Appoint a chairperson for each committee. Do not appoint the CCRM as the chairperson. Why not? After each member has completed the priority sheets, have the CCRM member of the group average the priority results. Now discuss and reprioritize this ranking as a group. Are prejudices involved in real life? Do managers really look at criteria in strict quantitative terms?
2. Visit a computer software vendor and ask for a copy of a recent response submitted to a RFP. Does the response follow the guidelines specified in the RFP? Does the vendor have a standard reporting format? Ask the vendor to share his or her thoughts on the various types of RFPs to which the vendor is asked to respond. Select four students to discuss their visits with vendors.

Suggested Readings

Austin, C.J. 1988. Informati*on systems for health services administration.* 3rd ed. Ann Arbor, MI: Health Administration Press.

Dorenfest, S.I., et al. 1987. *The state of the art in hospital information systems.* Northbrook, IL: Dorenfest & Associates.

Higgins, C.S., and R.E. Wilcox. 1989. *The health care directory.* North Easton, MA: Stonehill College.

Mandell, S.L. 1987. *Introduction to computers using the IBM and MS-DOS PCs with BASIC.* 2nd ed. St. Paul: West Publishing Co.

Packer, C.L. 1988. *Shared data research.* Hudson, OH.

Priest, S.L. 1982. *Managing hospital information systems.* Rockville, MD: Aspen Publishers.

Rowland, H.S., and B.L. Rowland. 1985. *Hospital software sourcebook.* Rockville, MD: Aspen Publishers.

Sneider, R.M. 1987. *Management guide to health care information systems*. Rockville, MD: Aspen Publishers.

Sneider, R.M. and P.F. Abrami. June 1985. Choosing the right information system for your hospital. *Healthcare Financial Management* 44–46.

Sullivan, D.R., T.G. Lewis, and C.R. Cook. 1986. *Using computers today with applications for the IBM PC*. Boston: Houghton Mifflin Co.

CHAPTER 5

Selecting Computer Resources

Introduction

The task of selecting computer resources such as microcomputers and application software from a multitude of vendors can be very complicated, confusing, and even frustrating. Each vendor may seem to have exactly what the organization needs with lists of references of satisfied customers who may be contacted to proclaim the success that can be achieved. Yet, is the vendor really the key to a satisfied user? Does a successful information system at one facility automatically guarantee success and satisfaction at another? How can one be sure that a vendor's promises will actually be met? Can the computer resource manager recommend and justify one vendor and system over another to a steering committee and users questioning why an equally qualified vendor was not chosen? Should the application software be developed, installed, and even programmed by the organization or acquired elsewhere? Various methods for evaluating these questions are discussed in this chapter.

There are several quantitative and subjective approaches to selecting computer resources and computer vendors (Austin 1988, Rowland and Rowland 1985). Whatever method is chosen, the selection should be made in a manner that minimizes the application bias of user areas and individuals and the individual preference for certain vendors, while still focusing on the computer resource objectives of the organization.

The selection of computer application and hardware resources begins with the preparation of a needs analysis, as presented in Chapter 4. This needs analysis is essential whether an organization will obtain the resources from vendors or other organizations or develop the system with an on-site staff. A needs analysis is essential even if the application or hardware is to be user-specific, as when acquiring a microcomputer and word processing software. Before one can select hardware and software, the user must know what is needed!

A request for proposal (RFP) includes the user and organization needs, a result of the need analysis. It is equally important that the vendor responses to the RFP be made in a format determined by the organization. Figures 4-10 through 4-15 are examples of reporting formats to which all vendors must respond. A reporting format permits side-by-side comparison of multiple vendors and eliminates the confusion of searching through cumbersome proposals for comparative data. There is minimal need to interpret vendor responses. For example, vendor pricing can be presented by rental cost, lease cost, purchase, and other combinations. These all represent various values of money and, to compare a multitude of vendors responding with different pricing schemes, one would have to interpret each vendor's proposal. Requiring all vendor responses to be in the same format minimizes user and staff interpretation of vendor proposals and quickly identifies proposals that have incomplete or missing responses. It also helps to ensure an "apples to apples" comparison.

Minicase 1: Frustrations of Vendor Selection

There are many examples of organizations being frustrated and indecisive in selecting vendors because the vendor submitted a standard proposal or a proposal that required extensive interpretations by the user. This can be avoided if a vendor's response to a RFP is in a predetermined format so that users will not second-guess whether they really understood what the vendor was offering. The following scenario actually happened: A RFP was sent to five vendors requesting proposals on software that could meet the need for an on-line patient registration system. The RFP did not require vendor responses to be in a specified format. The vendors responded with proposals that essentially were sales brochures and standard sample contracts containing quoted prices. It was necessary to interpret many of the vendor offerings. During separate interviews with each vendor, it became obvious that each vendor was offering a different flavor of response to the RFP, but the proposals could not easily be compared. However, one vendor who seemed to understand "best" what the organization wanted was finally selected. The vendor's standard contract was then signed.

The services and pricing that the vendor actually provided were entirely different from what was interpreted and presumed from the proposal. For example, the user began to receive invoices for all on-site microcomputer application training sessions. Indeed, this item was the organization's responsibility and was later noted by the vendor to be in their standard contract, but the user manager had never noticed or budgeted for these items. Training costs had been requested in the RFP, but the vendor's proposal did not respond to this request in a legible and quantitative manner. The manager had interpreted these costs as being included in the cost quotations. As the manager said, "It certainly appeared a very reasonable assumption that, when one buys software, how to use it should be part of that cost!" The budget was quickly exceeding cost estimates and the manager was placed in the embarrassing position of appearing to not fully comprehend the total costs of the project.

Other frustrating and unexpected situations arose for the manager. The RFP had stated that "... power requirements would be the same as present ..." yet, upon installation, the department was told by the vendor that additional power and environmental fixtures were necessary. Since the vendor's standard contract stated that the organization was responsible for environmental requirements, it had to absorb these unexpected costs even though the vendor's salesperson had "thought" that the present environment was sufficient. This situation could have been avoided by requiring the vendor to respond to the RFP specification in a format that addressed this specific need.

The vendor's installation analyst had been with the vendor only four months, was not completely trained in the system's operation, and had no previous health-care experience. This lack of health-care expertise resulted in the user manager having to design many of the screen entry formats. This was contrary to the verbal agreement between the salesperson and manager that the vendor would design the entry screens during installation and later provide on-site training for the user staff. This unplanned necessity for the user staff to design the screens resulted in extensive delays in installation because of the user staff's inexperience with the new system and its initial start-up and installation needs. This delay could have been avoided with a RFP that required an answer stating that the installation analyst would program the system as agreed to by the salesperson.

Other problems that surfaced during installation were inadequate user and technical manuals and the absence of mutually agreed-upon acceptance criteria between the organization and the vendor to ensure that the system's response time met the RFP-mandated response specifications. In addition, after two months of operation, the disk storage capacity was found to be inadequate because the vendor had recommended the wrong microcomputer capacity disk. The vendor had not done an in-depth analysis of the transaction volumes and storage needs.

Because the vendor's standard contract served as its proposal, the organization was faced with either complying with its set terms or attempting to invalidate the contract. By the time that the extent of the problem was recognized, the commitment to the project was such that the organization decided to continue the installation. The die was cast!

The frustrated user manager, whose credibility was being questioned by senior management and the steering committee, could have avoided this whole situation if a proper selection method and a specified contract negotiation process had been used.

When numerous vendors respond in a multitude of formats, the effort required to understand and compare each proposal can be extraordinary, and the assumptions generally inaccurate. The proposals will usually contain paraphernalia unrelated to the organization's specific needs. The proposals will include various pricing structures and additional system capabilities that will make it very difficult to compare each vendor's offerings with thc facilities' needs. Reviewing a voluminous proposal in search of a vendor's proposed delivery date can be time-consuming and often fruitless. Determining a proposed system's cost per patient visit can be exasperating, as well as usually being inaccurate, particularly if one has to interpret monthly lease costs, maintenance fees, one-time costs, manual update costs, and purchase costs. Furthermore, all of the cost proposals may not be for the same timeframe. For instance, one vendor might respond with annual costs and another with five-year costs. Most of these interpretations and inadequacies can be eliminated by requiring all vendor proposals to be in the same format.

Preliminary Compliance with the Request for Proposal

The purpose of a preliminary RFP screening method is to identify quickly vendors who should be eliminated from consideration, allowing the organization to focus attention upon candidates meeting minimal system and service requirements. An organization's RFP may result in a variety of vendor proposals. Some of these vendors will be serious candidates for consideration, whereas others either do not meet system requirements or do not have the ability to provide the needed scope of services.

As discussed earlier in this chapter, some vendors will submit standard proposals that do not conform to the organization's RFP response requirements. Some vendors will make a meek attempt to follow specifications, and others will submit their standard proposal and contract. These proposals usually demonstrate little concern for or understanding of the organization's needs and normally are cause for elimination of the vendor from further consideration. Other vendors will submit proposals that appear to conform to the RFP specifications, but in reality do not meet the organization's needs. Lastly, there are vendors who respond exactly as specified in the RFP and whose proposals deserve more thorough consideration.

The user and central computer resource managers must determine the requirements for a vendor to be considered for further review. The preliminary compliance checklist of Figure 5-1 is an example of criteria used to screen proposals for minimal requirements (Table 5-1). The list allows a quick evaluation of each proposal to determine the vendor's ability to meet the organization's main objectives.

Needless to say, the evaluation of vendor proposals requires a great deal of effort. It therefore is usually wise to restrict the number of RFPs sent out. A screening of potential vendors for such factors as time in business and number of clients will usually eliminate high risk vendors before the RFP is sent.

Figure 5-1. Checklist for preliminary proposal evaluation. Reprinted from *Managing Hospital Information Systems* by S. L. Priest, 1982, p. 66, with permission of Aspen Publishers, Inc.

	Vendor			
	A	B	C	D
1. Applications Proposed as Requested				
2. Component Descriptions & Performance				
3. Space & Site Requirements				
4. System Expansion Capabilities				
5. Applications Software Described				
6. Utilization Analyzed				
7. Input, Output, & Files Analyzed				
8. Delivery Schedule				
9. Support & Documentation Information				
10. Maintenance Information				
11. Annual Cost below $5.00 per Day.				
12. Training				

Rating Legend: C—Complete, IC—Incomplete, NA—Not Acceptable

Table 5-1. Preliminary Compliance Criteria.[a]

Evaluation Criteria	Vendor A	Vendor B	Vendor C	Vendor D	Vendor E
5-year cost					
— Hardware & software	$1,260,665	$3,916,961	$1,841,600	$1,901,973	$1,243,743
— Staffing	625,000	500,000	625,000	125,000	250,000
— Software from another vendor	0	225,000 (Lab)	0	225,000 (Lab)	50,000 (order entry)
	$1,885,665	$4,641,961	$2,466.600	$2,251,973	$1,543,743
Cost per patient day	$3.77	$9.28	$4.93	$4.50	$3.08
Physical renovations	major	major	major	minimum	minimum
Ease of implementation					
— User effort	major	moderate	major	moderate	moderate
— Computer resource staff effort	major	major	major	minimum	moderate
— Vendor effort	major	major	major	major	major
Demonstratable installations	2	2	56	over 210	over 200
Capacity for growth					
— Additional applications	in-house staff	vendor	in-house staff	vendor	in-house staff
— Additional volume	good	good	good	good	good

Table 5-1, continued.

Evaluation Criteria	Vendor A	Vendor B	Vendor C	Vendor D	Vendor E
Applications suitability — Missing applications — Adequacy of applications (INPAT REG, OPD REG, O.E. LAB, PHAR) (10 is maximum)	— 9, 7, 7, 8, 9	Lab 9, 9, 9, 0, 7	— 9, 9, 9, 9, 8	Lab 9, 9, 9, 0, 9	order entry 9, 9, 0, 9, 9
Proposal quality as one received	good	very good	poor	fair	fair
Consistency with recommended processing approach of distributed & turnkey	mainframe with limited turnkey	mainframe & turnkey	mainframe & turnkey	distributed	distributed
Financial system Interface	direct	tape	tape	tape	tape
Burden of success (user, vendor, shared between user and vendor)	user	user	user	shared between user	Mostly user, some shared
Stability of vendor	good	frequent change in personnel	frequent change in ownership	good	good

•Reprinted from *Managing Hospital Information Systems* by S. L. Priest, 1982, pp. 68–69, with permission of Aspen Publishers, Inc.

A multiphysician office selecting a billing and appointment system gives an example of preliminary selection criteria. If the office staff has no computer experience, it would not be appropriate to have the on-site staff be responsible for the installation of and training on the system. Extensive on-site vendor-provided training and overseeing is needed. The organization required that any vendor to be considered must be able, as a minimal criterion, to provide experienced staff on-site. Using this minimal selection requirement of on-site training and experienced staff, a vendor that submitted a proposal that required the organization's staff to install the system was automatically eliminated from further consideration.

Vendors who attempt to conform to the RFP specifications but have missing or ambiguous responses may be allowed to clarify these items within a set period and then, if no acceptable response is made, be eliminated from further consideration. Vendors should clarify responses not in conformance with the RFP specifications. Assumptions made by the organization may be inaccurate and lead to vendor and user disenchantment. For example, if a vendor responded to a requirement to submit five-year costs with a proposal that covered seven years, the organization should not have to interpret the costs to compare five years. The vendor must resubmit the response to conform to the RFP response specifications.

There are many ways to interpret questions, so the RFP should be as clear and specific as possible. One way to check the clarity of a question is to have a member of the staff try to answer the question.

When proposals from vendors are received, they should be perused for completeness, conformity to requested RFP formats, and reflection of an understanding of the organization's needs. Are references provided along with the number of years that each system has been installed? Are the proposed costs reasonable? Are the capacity and response-time estimates well-founded?

The vendor's costs should be competitive with other vendors' and be within the organization's budget. A vendor who submits a patient day cost of $0.50 when other proposals have costs of over $3.00 should be questioned as to what differences between this vendor and the competitor justify such large cost differences. Perhaps the RFP was misinterpreted or had essential items missing. Further, a vendor submitting a cost of $10 per day when other estimates are at $3.00 should be asked why the costs are so high.

The proposal should be examined for facility limitations. For instance, if the organization does not have space available for a large computer and a vendor requires an environmentally controlled and dedicated computer room and operations staff, this may immediately eliminate the vendor.

Thus, preliminary screening criteria identify those vendors who should clearly be eliminated from further consideration. The recommendations from the preliminary screening evaluation can be presented to the steering committee and others who have participated in the study for explanation, discussion, and concurrence. Vendors who have been eliminated should be sent a letter confirming their rejection, briefly stating the reason for the rejection, and thanking them for the proposal.

Vendor Presentations

Vendors to be considered further can make presentations to the steering committee, users, and other concerned individuals. Up to this stage of the evaluation process, the committee has generally been kept informed of the submissions and capabilities of the vendors by the central computer resources manager (CCRM). It is now time for the entire committee to meet the vendors. In addition, users not directly represented on the committee should be invited if they will be affected by the applications to be discussed. For instance, if a pharmacy system is to be discussed, a pharmacy representative, preferably the department head, should be invited to the presentations.

Each vendor should be given the same amount of time to make a presentation and answer committee questions. Before the meeting, each vendor should be informed of particular concerns of the committee. If the ability of the vendor to provide a particular application is questionable, the vendor must address that particular concern in the presentation, whereas another vendor may need to address its ability to interface its software with other vendors' applications.

Prior to the vendor presentations, the CCRM can prepare for the committee a vendor summary describing each vendor's conformity to the screening criteria, a brief background of the vendor, and other information necessary for the committee to prepare questions and concerns.

At the end of a presentation, the committee should meet and discuss its observations and concerns. The screening criteria of Figure 5-1 and Table 5-1 that were applied to each vendor may be used as the agenda for discussion. The CCRM should maintain the minutes of these meetings.

Reference Checks

Vendor reference checks to determine the validity of each proposal as well as the reputation and solvency of the vendor can begin before vendor meetings. User group organizations should be contacted. A vendor with an established user group (as described in Chapter 6) usually is an excellent source of reference lists of user organizations.

A vendor who refuses to provide a user list or supplies a partial list should be carefully screened, and the dependability and stability of the vendor should be questioned. Granted, all users may not be satisfied, but a vendor who circumvents questions about customers should be closely evaluated.

Reference checks should verify statements made in the proposal. The reference should confirm the existence of an application function and its conformance to RFP specifications. Do the vendor's application volume estimates and timings compare to what other users have found? Is the recommended implementation schedule reasonable, and do all performance claims agree with those obtained by the vendor's customers? Are the expansion and flexibility of the hardware and software consistent with the vendor claims? Essentially, all of the items in Figures 4-10 through 4-15 should be validated by contact with users of the system.

The vendor's financial stability can be reviewed through an audited financial statement. Frequently, vendors will offer comment on another vendor's stability and, although this may be just a sales ploy, it should be researched. Usually, the chief financial officer can assist with this function by reviewing financial reviews, such as Dun and Bradstreet reports, and contacting other users and even the vendor's bank for a financial rating.

The reference evaluation criteria listed in Table 5-2 are typical reference check areas that should be of concern to the organization. Again, these items may result in a decision for a vendor to be eliminated from further consideration. For instance, the reference check may show that, although the company has a systems support staff, they are inexperienced in health-care systems and thus many hours of the organization's own time will be required simply to educate the vendor on health-care terminology and needs.

Site Visits

Site visits can occur throughout the selection process. Before preparing the RFP, an organization may visit another facility to determine what it should include in its own RFP specifications and which vendors should receive the RFP. When the committee is in the final stages of determining finalist vendors, a site visit will again be essential.

Site visits relate to the "seeing is believing" evaluation that ensures confidence in final decisions. It is through visits to organizations using the vendor's proposed system that the committee and users experience the degree of services that a vendor is actually providing. A committee exposed only to written proposals, sales presentations, and other orientation sessions has essentially experienced the opinions of the vendor's idealized package. Through site visits, a steering committee can get first hand exposure to the vendor's proposed system. Site visits, if conducted properly, can provide valuable insights into a vendor's character and user commitment. Committee members can have many of their reservations cleared after viewing an installed system and discussing mutual concerns with peers.

Visits also provide the committee with an opportunity to interview people actually using the system. This will often reveal the feelings of the user for both the system and the vendor and also indicate what the role of the organization should be to ensure a successful installation. Site visits are not for learning how to use a vendor's system, but only for seeing how it works.

Both positive and negative comments during the visit can be informative. For example, one group made a site visit to view a registration and scheduling system. The user continually complained about the system, but not about the vendor. During the tour of the user area, it became clear that the reason for user dissatisfaction was not so much the system, but another user who was providing incomplete data into the system. Further, it was discovered that there was no interaction between the two users. The system was functioning as represented by the vendor, but the management of both areas refused to interact and used no audit techniques to maintain and monitor the system. When a visit was made to another organization with the same system, the committee found satisfied users and a system that was very efficient and contributed significantly to a well-run area.

Thus, site visits should be approached with an open mind. Each committee member should be cognizant of the fact that a successful system and vendor at one organization do not guarantee a success at one's own organization. It is generally users, not vendors, who make a successful system. Discussions with peers will help users clarify their roles and responsibilities regarding the CR.

There should be sufficient preparation before a site visit. The person setting up the site visit, the user computer resources manager (UCRM) or CCRM, should ensure that the site can demonstrate the needs of the organization and those addressed by the vendor in the proposal. Preferably, the site should be comparable in size and volume to the organization. It is a bad experience for a committee to visit a site and see an application that does not meet the committee's minimal expectations. This can result in a committee that has wasted a valuable day. Be sure to select the proper site for visiting.

Table 5-2. Reference evaluation criteria.

Selection Factor	Relative Weight	Factor Rating				Factor Score (Weight x Rating = Score)
		0	1	3	5	
Overall Organization Satisfaction		Totally unresponsive	Satisfied with at least two elements (service, support, equipment, and applications); no major impediments to user operations; reasonable cost	Satisfied with at least three elements (service, support, equipment, and applications); no major impediments to user operations; reasonable cost	Very satisfied with service, support, applications, and equipment; systems definitely enhance user operations at reasonable cost	
Overall Cost		Totally unresponsive	Cost quotes slightly exceeded, and per patient day costs somewhat above those for other organizations with comparable service	Cost quotes met and per patient day costs equal those for other organizations with comparable service	Cost quotes not exceeded and per patient day costs under those for other organizations with comparable service	
Vendor Responsiveness to Support and Installation		Totally unresponsive	Some significant delays with installation and difficulty in obtaining ongoing support (over 3 months late, 2-week wait)	Installation accomplished with minor delays and minor difficulty in obtaining ongoing support	Installation smooth with adequate ongoing support readily provided (on schedule, little or no wait)	

Table 5-2, continued.

Selection Factor	Relative Weight	Factor Rating				Factor Score (Weight x Rating = Score)
		0	1	3	5	
Maintenance Respon-siveness		Totally unresponsive	Frequent delays in providing, frequently exceeding time limit, plus some need for callback	Usually provided within stated time limits plus infrequent need for callback	Always provided within stated time limits and no need for callback	
Equipment Reliability		Totally unresponsive	Over 10% downtime	Between 5 and 10% downtime	Less than 5% downtime	
Availability of Applications		Totally unresponsive	Significant requested and important applications not available	Most requested and important applications available	All requested and important applications available	
Adequacy of Applications		Totally unresponsive	Significant deficiencies in meeting requested specifications and identified needs	Applications usually meet requested specifications and identified needs	Applications always meet requested specifications and identified needs	
Adaptability of Applications to user needs		Totally unresponsive	Applications infrequently adaptable to peculiar user needs	Applications usually adaptable to peculiar user needs	Applications always adaptable to peculiar user needs	
Adequacy of training		Totally unresponsive	Training only provided in basics	Training provided in most needed areas	Training provided in all needed areas	

Reprinted with permission of A. T. Kearney, Inc.

The committee should decide which members will make the visit. Preferably, people with the ability to understand the application fully should attend. It is not necessary for all committee members to go on all visits. If a laboratory system is viewed, there should be at least one person from the laboratory, preferably at least the UCRM, in attendance. A system that functions well in one organization may not conform to the needs of another facility. Often, this can only be determined by the potential user.

An overview of the organization to be visited should include such information as patient volumes, client load, physicians in the group and specialties, vendor applications being used, and the vendor features that will be seen. Figure 5-2 is a sample committee site visit ovcrvicw handout. The handout may also include samples of output reports and screens obtained from the vendor and site.

Everyone scheduled for the visit should meet beforehand to review what should be evaluated during the visit. This meeting allows the vendor's proposal to be reviewed by the committee. Also, the people most affected by the applications can be prepared to compare the required application features with the observed features.

In getting to the site, the group should travel together if possible. Informal, off-the-cuff conversation among the group is often invaluable for the visitors to understand each other's feelings and concerns.

When at the site, instead of immediately touring the area, there can first be a brief overview provided by the host. This will put into perspective the prior and postinstallation history of the applications and serve to inform the host of areas and users who are of particular concern to the group.

During the tour, there should be time arranged for each member to ask questions of his or her peers. For example, during a laboratory tour, the pathologist in the group will want to discuss particulars with the host pathologist. The same is true of laboratory supervisors. It is important for all members to learn the feelings of their counterparts.

One important goal of the visit should be to observe the attitude of the people responsible for using the application. It is important for the committee to develop an awareness of the user's attitude toward the system, while bearing in mind that attitude is a function of many things, including user competence. These observations will determine whether the vendor's representation is satisfactory to the host organization and what items the vendor may need to improve. The visit will also reveal whether the applications require unique controls as well as what the user must consider when planning for installation, staffing, training, and procedures that may need to be changed or added.

During the site visit, the detail of the vendor's applications should be reviewed and the length of time that the application has been in use should

Figure 5-2. Site visit overview handout. Reprinted from *Managing Hospital Information Systems* by S. L. Priest, 1982, p. 78, with permission of Aspen Publishers, Inc.

OUTLINE FOR SITE VISIT—NOVEMBER 12, 19__

STATISTICS: Beds—278 Employees—1044 Outpatient/ER visits annual—70,000 Percent Occupancy—93% Computer Vendor—XYZ

APPLICATIONS & FEATURES

IN AND OUT REGISTRATION
- Preadmissions
- Bed Availability
- Daily Admission/Discharges/Transfers
- Census Look-up
- Printing of Registration Forms
- Financial System Interface
- Demographic Recall for Outpatients and Assignment of Medical Record Number

PHARMACY
- Formulary
- Patient Profile
- Drug Schedule
- Label and Worksheet
- Dispensing Sheet for Nursing
- Dosage Calculation
- Drug Reaction/Interaction

VENDOR HARDWARE

	Visual Display Units	Printers
ER	14	1
Admitting	3	3
Medical Rec.	5	1
Laboratory	25	6
Pharmacy	13	4
Outpatient	11	2

LABORATORY
- Work Scheduling
- Patient Test Results
- Cumulative Results
- Q.C.
- Statistics (monthly)
- Monthly Discharge Cumulative Listing
- Outstanding Specimens
- Abnormals
- Specimen Drawing List
- Order Entry
- Test Result Entry
- Coulter S Interface
- Used in Chemistry, Bacteriology, Urology, Hematology, Microbiology
- Patient Test Results Available On-line in Emergency Room
- Financial System Interface

MEDICAL RECORDS
- Soundex Search
- Locator of Medical Record #

The above features can be seen at General Hospital. The systems do have additional features, but they are not used at the hospital.

AGENDA

8:30 a.m.	Leave hospital
10:00 a.m.	Mr. Smith, Vice-President, Computer Resources, will provide welcome and an overview of applications.
10:30 a.m.	We will break into two groups and tour each area listed above. Before viewing an area, the supervisor will provide a brief overview, answer questions, and be made aware of any particular concerns.
11:30 a.m.	Lunch and return to hospital thereafter.

be determined. If the pharmacy is not using the vendor's inventory function, perhaps this function is not usable because of unsatisfactory system design by the vendor or perhaps the pharmacy has other reasons. Thus, simply asking a host to explain his or her particular usage of a package may not be sufficient to determine the strengths and weaknesses of the complete package.

The organization should ask the host if the vendor meets delivery schedules and if user and technical manuals are available and routinely updated. The dependability of the equipment should be addressed for uptime and response time, and the hardware and software maintenance should be reviewed.

While at the site, the committee should explain to the host its RFP specifications and the vendor's responses to make sure that the vendor representation of a function conforms to that understood, and needed, by the user. The fact that a vendor has a laboratory reporting capability does not mean that this capability is what the organization requires. Questioning the host will usually provide insight into whether the functional capability is what the organization expects.

The questions in Figure 5-3 are samples of what can be asked of the hosts. In addition, a member of the group should maintain notes of the visit for later comparison with other visits and vendor representatives.

The site visit, if possible, should include a discussion with someone who had been involved in the host's prior method of operation. This person's comments and observations will be invaluable in the planning of realistic implementation schedules, training programs, and procedures and for other contingencies.

The return trip is an opportune time to get members' impressions of the site and vendor capabilities. These observations should also be included in the notes of the visit.

There is one minor problem with site visits, which is the time necessary to coordinate all of the people who must be consulted and to find a common day available for the visit. It may even take weeks before visits can be arranged, but the importance of these tours easily offsets the delays involved. It is important never to forget the scope of what is to be decided.

Quantitative Evaluations

The result of preliminary evaluation screening, vendor presentations, and site visits is usually the selection of one to three finalist vendors that the committee feels can meet the cost, service, and quality parameters for the organization's need. These processes have excluded vendors who initially

Figure 5-3. Site visit questions. Reprinted from *Managing Hospital Information Systems* by S. L. Priest, 1982, p. 78, with permission of Aspen Publishers, Inc.

1. Does the hardware/software vendor service the equipment/software promptly and effectively?
2. Does the equipment/software perform as specified in the proposal?
3. Was the equipment/software delivered on time and was the system installed on schedule?
4. Was adequate and high-quality training provided?
5. What particular problems or factors became of concern during implementation or ongoing operation?
6. Are the company's support people competent and able to work in harmony with your staff?
7. How did the conversion process go—smoothly, accurately, timely, etc.?
8. Were growth projections accurate with respect to equipment, software, and people needs?
9. What other companies were considered by your organization and why were they not selected?
10. Were there any hidden costs in the vendor's proposal that were discovered upon installation?
11. What would you do differently if you had the opportunity again?

appeared to meet the organization's needs but, upon closer investigation, did not have the ability or facilities to do so.

If the screening, presentations, and visits result in one finalist vendor, the decision has been made and is readily justified. If there are two or more finalists, a further, refined, quantitative approach can be used.

The usage of relative weights to give degrees of importance to certain selection criteria has often been questioned. Some people argue that weights are too subjective and result in just the opposite of the intended effect. Thus, some organizations simply use criteria that carry an equal weight with all concerns in order to judge and select a final vendor. However, the usage of relative weights should play an important role in the selection process. Although it is hard to dispute that weights are not subjective, they do allow the feelings of the committee and end-users to surface. This allows decisions to be made on items that really matter to the organization. An organization that has a proven development track record may not be so intent upon the vendor providing user training sessions and, conversely, an organization with an inexperienced staff may require the system to be installed by the vendor.

The underlying goals and objectives of individuals often surface with the use of weighted criteria. The question is how to develop true relative weights. When weights are the result of composite committee scores, they may not reflect the organization's true concern but only mask various feelings. The actual ranking factors can often only be decided at a committee meeting with an understanding of what each factor means and where each member can express his or her concerns.

Minicase 2: A Relative Weight Evaluation

An example of relative weight usage in an organization follows. To establish a reliable basis for vendor comparison, one utilizes a method of assigning values of relative weight. Some main criteria can be selected by the committee. In this case the following five major categories were used: hardware, software, equipment costs, support capabilities, and other factors.

Under each major category, a number of questions were applied to each vendor's proposal. The questions were included in the RFP for vendor response. The questions were tailored to the specific needs of the organization. Each proposal was evaluated in light of these needs, and each response was assigned a numerical value of 1 through 5, with 5 being the most favored position. For those categories where two or more vendors were thought to be equal, a value of 3 was assigned. The values were subtotaled for each vendor by major category and then combined to arrive at a total raw score by vendor, as shown in Table 5-3.

Each major category was assigned a weighting factor to give value to its relative importance in the overall evaluation. These factors were developed by the steering committee before vendor proposals were reviewed. The weights ranged from 1 through 10, with 10 being the most important.

Each weighting factor was applied to the major category subtotal for each vendor so that an appropriate total weight score could be derived, as shown in Table 5-4. The resulting weighted totals for all vendors presented a better representation of the relative merits of each proposal.

Table 5-3. General Organization Vendor Ranking.

Criteria Categories	**Vendor**		
	A	**B**	**C**
Hardware			
Variety of peripherals	3	3	3
Through-put capability	4	4	5
Adequacy for present needs	3	2	3
Adequacy for future needs	3	2	4
How long operational?	5	5	3
Back up capabilities	3	3	3
Redundancy	5	3	3
Upgrading ease	3	3	4
	29	25	28
Software			
Period operational	4	4	3
Easily modified	3	3	3
Adequacy	3	3	3
Utility routines available	3	3	3
Operating System available	3	3	4
Medical service packages	3	3	4
Application timing	3	3	4
Available languages	2	3	4
	24	25	28
Equipment costs			
Best lease	3	4	5
Base use hours-lease	2	4	3
Additional overtime	2	4	4
Best purchase	2	3	3
Best maintenance	3	4	5
Cost of communications	2	3	4
	14	22	24
Support capabilities			
Schools—type/location	2	5	3
Systems assistance	3	4	3
Field engineering	3	4	3
Preinstallation test time	4	4	3
Preventive maintenance	3	3	4
	15	20	16
Other factors			
Proposal quality	3	4	5
Vendor experience	4	3	4
Confidence level	2	3	3
User references	3	3	4
Cost of recording media	4	4	3
	16	17	19
Total raw score	101	113	120

Table 5-4. Weighted vendor rankings.

		Vendor		
Major Category	**Weight**	**A**	**B**	**C**
Hardware	8	256	232	264
Software	7	168	175	196
Equipment costs	10	140	220	240
Support capabilities	7	105	140	112
Other factors	5	80	85	95
Weighted totals		749	852	907

This method of evaluation does not provide full justification for the final selection, but rather furnishes a means of ranking each vendor in relation to the others on an overall basis. One must realize, in the attempt for purely "objective" quantitative analysis, that some vendors are more honest and up front than others. Appropriate subjective management concerns must clearly be applied in addition to these values before the final selection. Tables 5-5 and 5-6 offer other cost, service, and application software quality criteria.

Forced Rankings

Another method that could be used in selecting a vendor is "forced ranking." For example, if five vendors are being considered there are five weights for cost. The vendor with the highest cost would be ranked number five and the others would be ranked appropriately. Ties would be permissible. Thus, the addition of the ranks as shown in Table 5-7 would serve to determine the final rank of the vendors, with the lowest point score demonstrating the most favored vendor.

Often this method reveals a vendor who is consistently number one, and no further evaluation is necessary. As with the relative weight approach, the forced ranking method allows members' feelings to surface and, even if one finalist vendor is not selected, can be instrumental in the final decision-making process.

Negotiating the Contract

The signing of a contract for computer resources enters the organization into a legal and financial commitment. Vendors are professional negotiators and make their living at it, whereas the CCRM and UCRMs often have neither legal background nor negotiating experience. For this reason, negotiations are usually handled by a negotiating team. Unless a member of senior management is an excellent negotiator, an outside counsel should be hired to lead the negotiations.

Some vendors, particularly the larger firms, have standard contracts that they deem to be nonnegotiable. This means that modification of the standard vendor contract is not a simple process and usually requires a combination of legal and computer expertise. However, if the vendor wants your business badly enough, almost anything can be negotiated in a contract. Telephone calls to a variety of known users will identify the extent to which contract changes have been negotiated.

Vendors frequently ask organizations to sign standard contracts. One should be extremely wary of this without first having the contract reviewed for both legal and technical contents. In fact, if at all possible the organization should draw up the contract for the vendor to sign! The vendor's own standard contract language can be incorporated in the contract, but in such a manner that the organization's needs are protected first.

It is better to get a vendor to change *your* contract, rather than theirs. Vendors usually have standard sales contracts that secure maximal protection for the vendor while providing the organization with minimal legal contract requirements.

Oral representations and demonstrations of a vendor's product are frequently different from that described in the final vendor proposed sales contract. There can also be a difference between the vendor's written response to the organization's RFP and the actual contract later presented for signature. Generally, no agreement made between the facility and vendor will be enforceable in a court of law unless it is specifically included in the final written contract.

During the initial discussions with the vendor, one should maintain an accurate record of all representations made by the vendor. This record can be included in the final contract.

Before signing a contract, one should thoroughly understand the commitments made by the vendor and the organization. The language of the contract is often in terms only an experienced computer-oriented lawyer can interpret. Further, the financial terms of the contract may not always be the most optimal for the organization. To ensure a contract that protects the organization, the organization's attorney should first review all legally

Table 5-5. Computer/systems selection weighted cost evaluation criteria.[a]

Selection Factor	Relative Weight[b]	Factor Rating				Factor Score (Weight x Rating = Score)
		0	1	2	3	
Cost Equipment		Totally unresponsive	Will cost more than $3.00 per patient day (1st year)	Will cost between $2.00 and $2.99 per patient day (1st year)	Will cost less than $2.00 per patient day (1st year)	
Hardware Maintenance		Totally unresponsive	Will be charged significantly above equipment costs	Will be charged somewhat above equipment costs	Included in equipment cost	
Software Maintenance		Totally unresponsive	Will be charged significantly above applications costs	Will be charged somewhat above equipment or applications costs	Included in applications costs	
Operating Software		Totally unresponsive	Will be charged significantly above equipment or applications cost	Will be charged somewhat above equipment or applications costs	Included in equipment or applications costs	
Inpatient Admitting		Totally unresponsive	Will cost more than $2.50 per patient day (5th year)	Will cost between $2.00 and $2.99 per patient day (5th year)	Will cost less than $2.00 per patient day (5th year)	

Table 5-5, continued.

Selection Factor	Relative Weight[b]	Factor Rating				Factor Score (Weight x Rating = Score)
		0	1	2	3	
Outpatient Registration/ Scheduling		Totally unresponsive	Will cost more than $2.50 per patient day (5th year)	Will cost between $1.50 and $2.49 per patient day (5th year)	Will cost less than $1.50 per patient day (5th year)	
Order Entry/ Charge Collection		Totally unresponsive	Will cost more than $1.50 per patient day (5th year)	Will cost between $1.00 and $1.49 per patient day (5th year)	Will cost less than $1.00 per patient day (5th year)	
Pharmacy		Totally unresponsive	Will cost more than $1.50 per patient day (5th year)	Will cost between $1.00 and $1.49 per patient day (5th year)	Will cost less than $1.00 per patient day (5th year)	
Laboratory Reporting		Totally unresponsive	Will cost more than $1.50 per patient day (5th year)	Will cost between $1.00 and $1.49 per patient day (5th year)	Will cost less than $1.00 per patient day (5th year)	
Training		Totally unresponsive	Will cost more than $5,000	Will cost less than $5,000	Included in equipment or application cost	

Table 5-5, continued.

Selection Factor	Relative Weight[b]	Factor Rating				Factor Score (Weight x Rating = Score)
		0	1	2	3	
Installation and Assistance		Totally unresponsive	Will provide less than 30 staff days at no charge	Will provide 30–60 staff days at no charge	Will provide whatever required to install and adapt system at no charge	
Personnel		Totally unresponsive	Will cost more than $2.00 per patient day (5th year)	Will cost between $1.00 and $1.99 per patient day (5th year)	Will cost less than $1.00 per patient day (5th year)	
Site Preparation		Totally unresponsive	Will cost more than $50,000	Will cost between $10,000 and $49,000	Will cost less than $10,000	
Five-Year Total Cost		Totally unresponsive	Will cost more than 2.0 million	Will cost between $1.5 million and $2.0 million	Will cost less than $1.5 million	

[a]Reprinted with permission of A. T. Kearney, Inc.
[b]Relative weights: 5, critical; 3, important; 1, significant.

Table 5-6. Weighted service and application evaluation criteria.[a]

Selection Factor	Relative Weight	Factor Rating				Factor Score (Weight x Rating = Score)
		0	1	2	3	
Equipment/ Applications Delivery		Totally unresponsive	Will require more than 6 months after final contract	Will require between 3 and 6 months after final contract	Will require less than 3 months after final contract	
Equipment Capacity and Growth Potential		Totally unresponsive	Capable of processing 60% of applications and no need for upgrade for 2 years	Capable of processing 80% of applications and no need for upgrade for 3 years	Capable of processing 95% of requested applications, and no need for upgrade for 5 years	
Availability of Backup Equipment/ Service		Totally unresponsive	Accessible and within 50 miles	Accessible and within 25 miles	Accessible and within 10 miles	
Level of Installation/ Support Assistance		Totally unresponsive	Only installation assistance provided at no charge; adequate vendor resources available within 2 weeks	Installation assistance and minimal ongoing support at no charge, adequate vendor resources available within 1 week	As much as required to fully install and operate the system at no charge	

Table 5-6, continued.

Selection Factor	Relative Weight[a]	Factor Rating				Factor Score (Weight x Rating = Score)
		0	1	2	3	
Level of Training		Totally unresponsive	All training chargeable, but responsive to basic needs	Installation training at no charge; other training available, and responsive to most needs	As much as required to fully install and operate the system at no charge	
User Manuals and Documentation		Totally unresponsive	Systems only	Systems and limited user manuals	Both systems and user manuals available	
Availability of Inpatient Admitting Software/ Applications		Totally unresponsive	60% of systems available	80% of systems available	All systems available	
Adequacy of Inpatient Admitting Software/ Applications		Totally unresponsive	60% of systems available as specified (absolute reports/feature)	80% of systems available as specified (absolute reports/feature)	All systems available as specified (absolute reports/feature)	
Availability of Outpatient Reg./ Schd. Software/ Applications		Totally unresponsive	60% of systems available	80% of systems available	All systems available	

Table 5-6, continued.

Selection Factor	Relative Weight	Factor Rating				Factor Score (Weight x Rating = Score)
		0	1	2	3	
Adequacy of Out-patient Reg./ Schd. Software/ Applications		Totally unresponsive	60% of systems available as specified (absolute reports/ features)	80% of systems available as specified (absolute reports/ features)	All systems available as specified (absolute reports/feature)	
Availability of Order Entry/Charge Collection		Totally unresponsive	Limited system available		All systems available as specified (absolute reports/feature)	
Availability of Order Entry/ Charge Collection		Totally unresponsive	Limited system available		Complete system available	
Adequacy of Order Entry/Charge Collection		Totally unresponsive	System only available for individual departments/ applications		System available throughout as appropriate	
Pharmacy Availability		Totally unresponsive	60% of systems available	80% of systems available	All systems available	

Table 5-6, continued.

Selection Factor	Relative Weight	Factor Rating				Factor Score (Weight x Rating = Score)
		0	1	2	3	
Pharmacy Adequacy		Totally unresponsive	60% of systems available as specified (absolute reports/ features)	80% of systems available as specified (absolute reports/ features)	All systems available as specified (absolute reports/feature)	
Laboratory Availability		Totally unresponsive	60% of systems available	80% of systems available	All systems available	
Laboratory Adequacy		Totally unresponsive	60% of systems available as specified (absolute reports/feature)	80% of systems available as specified (absolute reports/feature)	All systems available as specified (absolute reports/feature)	
Amount of Preventive Maintenance		Totally unresponsive	More than 4 hours/month required (prime time)	2 to 4 hours/month required (non-prime time)	No more than 2 hours/ month required (non-prime time)	
Response of Breakdown Maintenance		Totally unresponsive	More than 8 hours, but less than 24 hours normal	2 to 8 hours normal	Less than 2 hours normal	

Table 5-6, continued.

Selection Factor	Relative Weight	Factor Rating				Factor Score (Weight x Rating = Score)
		0	1	2	3	
Adherence to RFP Format and Specifications		Totally unresponsive	Sizable deviations from format and specifications (60–90% adherence)	Generally adhered to format and specifications (90%)	Total adherence to RFP format and specifications	

[a]Reprinted with permission of A.T. Kearney, Inc.

Table 5-7. Forced rankings of vendors.[a]

Criteria	Vendor A	Vendor B	Vendor C	Vendor D	Vendor E
Cost per patient day	1	4	3	2	5
Early delivery date	2	5	4	1	2
Number of proven installations	1	3	5	2	4
Additional staffing	1	2	3	2	4
Ease of user use	2	3	4	4	1
Level of training	1	5	3	2	5
Total	8	22	22	13	21

[a]Key: 1—vendor has most favorable proposal; 2—vendor has second most favorable proposal; 3—vendor has third most favorable proposal; 4—vendor has fourth most favorable proposal; 5—vendor has fifth most favorable proposal.

binding contracts. Preferably, potential negotiating team members would be an attorney with knowledge of computer contracts, a financial officer, a purchasing agent, the central computer resource manager, the chief operating officer, and even a technical consultant to the organization.

The CCRM and technical consultant can provide the negotiating team with the reasons for and the requirements of the acquisition and can suggest negotiable items such as delivery, acceptance criteria, ongoing performance criteria, etc. The legal counsel can ensure the proper wording and scope of the contract and clarify the purpose and limits of each item in the contract. Often, postinstallation problems such as inadequate training can be traced to ambiguities in or omissions from the formal agreement, which can be prevented with proper legal counsel. The CCRM and counsel must work together for completeness of the contract and ensure that all issues are addressed.

The purchasing department will provide negotiating skills and ensure maximal concern with length of warranty, penalties, and other matters of routine to an experienced purchasing agent. The financial officer can provide the best methods of financing the acquisition and will ensure that the contract cost terms are appropriate.

The chief operating officer (COO) will provide assurance that the contract is consistent with organization goals and objectives. The COO also provides the support and backing of the entire organization. The presence of this person minimizes any question about what the CR acquisition represents to the organization.

When negotiating a contract, the team should have a prioritized list of items that should be addressed in the contract. The list should include all major objectives such as acceptance criteria parameters, maintenance warranties, cost limits for vendor charges, and delivery standards. This priority list should be openly discussed among team members before meeting with the vendor.

Various negotiating strategies should be decided upon by the negotiation committee. Frequently, a number of informal negotiating sessions may occur before the vendor's decision-making authority is known. Time can be saved if the vendor's contract signer is identified at the onset of negotiations. If possible, one should only negotiate with a vendor representative who can make decisions, preferably the person who will sign the contract. Nothing is more frustrating than dealing with a salesperson who has to return later with an acceptance or rejection of negotiated terms.

Literature sources deal with general and specific clauses that must be considered when negotiating a contract (Memel and Sherwin 1988, Nimmer 1985). These items will not be detailed here. A checklist should be followed to ensure proper consideration of all items. Items on the list might include: documentation manuals, payment terms, performance standards, corrections to software or hardware, what happens to the equipment and software if the vendor goes out of business, and what would be cause for a right to cancel.

Usually, standard software contracts address the legal aspect of granting the usage of the equipment or software, warranty and liability of the vendor for consequential damages, and the organization service items such as maintenance, training, program enhancements, etc. It is in the area of vendor services that terms can most generally be negotiated: number of support days, payment terms, length of warranty period, and updates to the software at no cost.

The contract should state the standard that will be used to measure the performance of a program or hardware, such as response time and storage capacities. Without such a standard, any program delivered by the vendor that conforms to the general description of the processing requirements will usually be deemed by the vendor to satisfy its obligation. To avoid future problems, the organization should incorporate any agreements, including software specifications, into the written contract. These can include future software changes necessary to meet legal requirements such as mandated Medicare reporting requirements. These processing requirements should also include definitions of the item, as various terms can mean different things to different people.

One method of providing a degree of vendor response to hardware problems may be to negotiate into the contract the requirement that the cost of systems and hardware maintenance be a function of the system's uptime. For instance, if the system can be used only 85% of its normally scheduled time, for reasons of downtime caused by hardware malfunctions and vendor response or repair persons, the monthly payment for this item would be only 85% of the normal bill. Hence, the organization will pay only for services rendered, and the vendor will have some degree of incentive for ensuring the maximal uptime of the hardware and operating software.

The instability of the software industry is a major area of concern. There is little capital investment needed to develop software, and the organization must protect itself in case the vendor goes out of business. The contract should cover nonperformance in case the package does not work as represented or if the company goes out of business. There must be clear title to the organization in this case. Further, payment terms may be arranged to pay only for progress that is accomplished. This provides an incentive for the vendor to remain on schedule. In extreme cases it may prevent the vendor's disappearance before the work is completed. When signing a contract, it is important to detail what the organization is receiving, who owns the software, and who maintains and updates the software.

The organization must be assured of the availability of the vendor in the foreseeable future if its software is to be vendor-serviced. At a minimum the contract should state that the package should be corrected by the vendor if errors are found or if the package does not perform as represented. The application package should always be demonstrated before negotiations begin. In addition, if the vendor does not provide the source code directly to the buyer, the organization needs the security of having the source code readily available, and it will be essential to include in the contract that the source code will be held in escrow by a third party, such as a bank.

The contract should clearly let the organization know what it will be receiving from the vendor. However, there are several points of view as to whether the complete request for proposal (RFP) should be included in the contract. Some RFPs contain a statement that the RFP will be part of the final contract. This, supposedly, tells the vendors that they will be held responsible for statements made in their proposals, so that hardware and software requirements and associated costs accurately reflect what the organization will be receiving. The argument against including the RFP in the contract is that the RFP may be very cumbersome—several hundred pages in length—and it is questionable as to whether each line is a legal commitment.

There is the possibility that just essential parts of the proposal—the application features and performance criteria—should be incorporated. However, many items in the RFP may not be completely appropriate to the final negotiations as the vendor may not have all of the features desired in an application. In this case only those items that the organization will be receiving should be included.

The organization must hold the vendor responsible for everything contained in the response to the request for proposal. After all, it was the vendor's proposal that was a main factor in selecting the vendor.

Minicase 3: The Contract for Results Reporting

The reasons to include the vendor response to RFP specifications in the contract can be seen in the following example. A manager had asked a potential vendor if the proposed software package would feature the storage and retrieval of patient test results. The vendor's proposal acknowledged that the feature was available as part of the proposal. After the contract was signed, without including the RFP specifications concerning test results, it was seen that the results were indeed stored, but were not capable of being retrieved in chronological order or by department, as had been presented in the vendor's proposal. If a nurse or physician wanted to look at laboratory BUN test results, all of the patients' results had to be scanned to locate the BUN. The clinical user had been led to believe by the vendor's proposal that the result feature was available, but the actual feature did not conform to the clinical needs. Had the RFP proposal specifications been required in the final contract, the vendor would have been more cautious about how its product was represented.

Signing the Final Contract

The final contract should cover all major risks and clearly set forth the intent of both parties. This will help in the case of a situation that is not covered explicitly in the contract. Many contracts have a clause addressing arbitration. Soma (1983) is one reference for sample contracts.

When discussing price, look for all maximal discounts offered by the vendor such as retroactive discounts and payment within 30 days. Further, it may be better not to accept a package price, but to get a breakdown of hardware and software components. A breakdown of items may reveal negotiable alternatives such as components that can be eliminated or downgraded while additions can be included without a price increase.

Once a contract is signed, one's attention should then be directed toward working cooperatively with the vendor. A competent vendor has a reputation to maintain and wishes to enhance that reputation with a successful installation. One should only have to refer to the contract when a major disagreement occurs and not for easily compromised problems.

Further, if the previously mentioned method for obtaining reference criteria was followed, the reaction of the vendor to user needs should already be known.

Selecting Microcomputer Software and Hardware

The selection concepts discussed in this chapter certainly apply to selecting microcomputer hardware and software. However, the selection of microcomputers and accompanying software takes less effort and time. Because the investment in microcomputer hardware and software is relatively small, users often take the selection process lightly. Microcomputers are generally perceived as having less of an impact outside of the immediate user area, yet the information processed can be vital to an organization.

In truth, the degree of selection effort and time depends on how the hardware and software will be used. The selection of a microcomputer for word processing may be different than that of a microcomputer that will run a database package for multiple users.

The perception is that microcomputer needs are obvious and that one does not need to go through a rigid needs definition and comparison process. One simply "goes out" and buys a microcomputer. This approach has left many users frustrated when they buy a microcomputer that cannot be fixed if broken, that will not run needed software, and for which they have no training on applications and operation.

One needs to operate within the scope of an organization microcomputer policy, as discussed in Chapter 10. Standardization, user-friendliness, local support and training, and staff and hardware backup are essential concerns when selecting microcomputers and software. In addition, there are a number of activities necessary before one commits to a particular brand and model of microcomputer hardware and software. The following can serve as guidelines when selecting a user-managed microcomputer. These guidelines can be tailored to meet individual user needs.

Software

A frequent approach is to buy the microcomputer first and then get the software. As with larger computers, the software should be the first and major consideration.

Does the software package have the capability you need? List these needs on paper and check them off in comparison to the software you are considering. Ask for a demonstration, as "seeing is believing." Make a site visit to an experienced user to see the package used in a manner similar to how you anticipate using it. Note the hardware and operating system it runs on and the specifications of the hardware (i.e., memory size, disk drive type, printer make and model).

Has the software been widely sold? Does your seller understand the software? Do not help the developer "debug" the software unless you are truly prepared for that approach. Hours upon hours are needed to debug software and then testing must be repeated once the corrections have been made.

Is the operating system an established system? Does your package run on it?

Is the software "user-friendly"? If you cannot learn to use the package in a matter of hours, chances are that a better package can be found.

Is the documentation adequate? Read it! Can you understand it?

Hardware

Will the software you need run on the hardware under consideration? Remember that most software for microcomputers runs on a certain brand of microcomputer and under a certain operating system.

Are there sufficient processing and storage capacity to meet your present requirements and sufficient expansion capacity to meet future needs?

How will repairs be made? If you do not buy the microcomputer locally, you will need to travel a distance to have it repaired. It may even be necessary to mail the microcomputer. Can you survive weeks without the system?

How established is the brand that you are considering? Remember, "pound wise, penny foolish." Microcomputer manufacturers have had a history of going out of business. Will this seller be here tomorrow for service and repairs?

Who will be training your staff? You? The seller? Remember the concerns about seller history.

If you plan to communicate with another computer, can it be done? Get a demonstration.

Do you expect more than one person to use the microcomputer at the same time? If yes, can the hardware handle this? Get a demonstration. What is the additional cost in terms of money and response time?

Does the quote from the seller include all that you need to make the system functional? Check that the system includes a printer, monitor, cables, and hard disk drives.

Let the Buyer Beware

An example of the wrong way to acquire a microcomputer is when one simply buys the hardware because it is on sale. Parents frequently buy a computer for their student with the perception that all microcomputers are alike. They do not take the time to ask what kind of microcomputer is used at the student's school. It is necessary to ensure that the student can use the same software at home as at school. Getting a good buy on a microcomputer does nothing for a student who cannot use the same software as at school.

Conclusion

The selection of computer resources and vendors represents a significant investment of time and money for the organization and can have a direct effect on the organization's routine operations. Perhaps 2 to 3% of an organization's finances will be directed to computer resources (Dorenfest et al. 1987). Most areas of the organization will become dependent on the resources in terms of both staff utilization and output. Systems that are cost-effective, enhance the quality of services, and complement a decision-making process will promote user confidence and commitment. To select the appropriate CRs, an organization uses quantitative and subjective methods to identify and account for all concerns.

The user faced with the selection of both multiple information systems and vendors has to weigh carefully the many choices available and consider these in conjunction with the CR sophistication of user and CR staff within the organization. Concerns as to whether an application should be installed by the user staff or provided from another source must be carefully weighed in terms of cost, staff, experience, and time.

An effective evaluation process usually begins with the preparation of a Request for Proposal (RFP), as discussed in Chapter 4. This allows the executive to compare various vendor proposals against established criteria that reflect the strengths and weaknesses of both the organization and the considered vendors. A selection method includes a preliminary screening phase during which essential criteria are used to screen vendors for more serious and intensive review. Reference checks and site visits can be used to determine the vendor's history of providing complete and accurate proposals and systems.

There are various quantitative methods that can be considered to select computer resources. One method is to use weighting factors for selected criteria. Another method force-ranks the vendors against each other.

Some people feel that weighting and ranking factors are arbitrary and, in fact, they are, especially when you begin questioning why one vendor gets one point and another gets three points for the same function. Scoring gives a committee a basis for a decision, however, by allowing the committee to quantify its desires and impressions.

In this chapter, the contract negotiation process and its role in the selection of a CR were reviewed briefly. The contract discussion is in no way complete and, before a contract is negotiated, the organization should contact legal counsel for guidance and assistance on the contract negotiating team.

Quantitative methods, however, are not the ultimate decision-making factors. They usually are only guidelines. Throughout the evaluation process, the committee and executive must express their feelings on all vendor offerings and concerns. Based on these discussions and on scores, the committee is able to make its decision.

The acquisition of a microcomputer begins with the software. The needs identification stage must be done first, and then the needs are compared with what the software offers. This can be done with site visits and demonstrations. The next step is to ensure that the software runs on the considered microcomputer and operating system. The hardware acquired must be complete as seen during the site visit and demonstration. The last step is to confirm the competence and track record of the seller.

Chapter 9 describes how one organization used the selection approaches addressed in this chapter.

Questions and Assignments

1. John Smith, M.D., has a home computer of brand Z. He uses brand X word processing software. It is well known in the office that Dr. Smith is microcomputer-literate. John Jones is the office manager of Dr. Smith's group practice. Mr. Jones has been asked to coordinate a computer selection committee to select a microcomputer and software that will do transaction billing for the physicians as well as other financial ledger tasks. A word processing package is also to be selected.

   The selection process discussed in this chapter identifies the "gut feeling" aspect of selecting computer resources after the quantitative process has been exhausted. The quantitative process has shown that brand Y microcomputer and brand S word processing software clearly meet the needs of the group practice. These are not the same microcomputer and word processing software that Dr. Smith is using. How do you carry out the final selection process? Discuss your reasoning.

2. One member of a computer selection committee has little knowledge of computer applications and usage. This person is easily swayed by the persuasiveness of the person addressing him. He cannot perceive how the committee's choice of vendor will meet his department's software needs. Other vendors seem to offer similar solutions—what is best for his department? Can you recommend an approach to ensure the member's support of the majority's choice? Do organization needs differ from department needs?

3. You have just completed a class in computer literacy. A friend approaches you and asks you to recommend the "one" best microcomputer. What is your advice?

Suggested Readings

Austin, C.J. 1988. *Information systems for health services administration.* 3rd ed. Melrose Park, IL: Health Administration Press.

Dorenfest, S.I., et al. 1987. *The state of the art in hospital information systems.* Northbrook, IL: Dorenfest & Associates, Ltd.

Memel, J.D., and L. Sherwin. January/February 1988. Winning in contract negotiations. *Healthcare Executive* (1):26–29.

Nimmer, R.T. 1985. *The law of computer technology*. Boston: Warren, Gorham and Lamont.

Priest, S.L. 1982. *Managing hospital information systems*. Rockville, MD: Aspen Publishers.

Rowland, H.S., and B.L. Rowland. 1985. *Hospital software sourcebook.* Rockville, MD: Aspen Publishers, 63–71.

Soma, J.T. 1983. *Computer technology and the law*. Colorado Springs, CO: Shepard's/McGraw-Hill.

CHAPTER 6

The Computer System Life Cycle

Introduction

A computer system is the integration of five components: computers (hardware), people, programs (software), procedures, and data. For example, a laboratory computer system is composed of visual display terminals (VDTs), printers, and a computer processor; laboratory staff such as technicians and pathologists; application programs; user policies and procedures; and data that are stored, updated, and retrieved in various manners. Without all five components functioning, the task—i.e., the processing and preparation of laboratory information—cannot be accomplished. Thus, a computer system is like a chain that is only as strong (as functional) as its weakest link.

System Life Cycle

A system life cycle (SLC) is a step-by-step breakdown of each phase of computer system development and installation into steps of manageable size. The process allows one to identify manageable components of the computer system. The SLC includes methods of identifying, designing, implementing, and maintaining a computer system. The SLC requires the participation of end-users, senior management, and the CRs staff. Developing a SLC can be an exciting and creative process that brings significant changes in user and organizational process. Without the SLC, one has a high probability of failure, frustration, and undue expense. The SLC must be understood and managed. The approach used to define and implement a computer system is as essential as the computer system itself. The success, scope, and usability of a computer system depend on following the SLC process.

The SLC provides the technique necessary for a computer system to evolve and grow. Each phase of the SLC is essential for the success of the system.

The SLC phases are (1) the inception phase, when an idea to use or enhance a computer system to meet the strategic and operational objectives of the organization is first presented; (2) the feasibility phase, when the decision of whether to implement the system is made; (3) the systems analysis phase, which provides detail and definition of the current process and where alternative solutions are offered; (4) the design phase, which includes specifications and decisions of whether to develop the application in-house or acquire it through vendors; (5) the training, conversion, and implementation phase, when the system is installed; (6) the ongoing phase, with maintenance and control; and (7) the postimplementation study phase to acknowledge the benefits of the computer system. These seven phases complete the SLC (Table 6-1). Further enhancements, changes, and even retirement of the computer system return the process to the inception phase and the SLC starts again.

The SLC requires (1) policies for computer system initiation, (2) the establishment of a work committee, (3) the participation in a user group, (4) security and confidentiality of computer resources, and (5) conversion and control techniques. The phases of the SLC are not dependent upon whether the computer resources (CRs) are managed by end-users or the central CR staff. The phases must be followed in varying degrees to ensure a high quality, long-term, successful computer resource.

Documentation

Each phase of the SLC produces documentation: written or pictorial reports describing what has taken place during that phase. This documentation allows management review to determine whether the system should proceed to the next phase. It also lets everyone involved with a phase know what is expected from them.

The SLC provides reference points to determine whether the computer system is on schedule and within costs and whether it will meet the ongoing needs of the end-users. The SLC process ensures that the computer system has been well thought out and that unforeseen and unplanned items are eliminated or at least minimized. It ensures that all concerns have been addressed, and it ensures a proper sequence of process and planning.

Table 6-1. Computer systems life cycle.

Stage	User	CR Staff	Steering Committee	Documentation
Inception	Initiate project	Preliminary survey Alternatives		Project Request Form
Feasibility	Evaluate existing system	Assist user Alternatives	Status	Feasibility report Status report
Systems analysis	Describe existing system Collect data Identify needs Select vendor	Assist user Select vendor	Approve request Prioritize Funding/staff	Requirements report Request for Proposal (RFP) Program specifications
System development	Approve plan		Status update	Status report
Training, conversion and installation	Training Testing	Assist user Coordinate implementation	Status update	Training schedule Implementation plan Instruction manuals
Operations	Monitor usage	Monitor	Status update	Operational reports
Postimplementation studies	Acknowledge benefits	Follow-up study	Status update	Follow-up report

Inception

Project Request Form

The first phase of the SLC begins when an end-user has an idea for a new or enhanced computer system stimulated by a need to improve information processing procedures. The idea is submitted to the CR staff via a project request form similar to Figure 6-1. Written requests for the utilization of computer resources, whether located within the user area or requiring CR staff, should be submitted on the form. The form ensures that some thought has been given to the project and its potential benefits.

A strange phenomenon can occur with project request forms. Over half of the forms distributed are NEVER returned! The implication is that over half of the projects requested via telephone or in hallways do not represent serious requests. The person making the request solved the problem while filling out the form, had little time for the necessary interaction described in Chapter 3, or realized later that the request was not feasible or was more involved than first believed. Documentation of the request is the first step in the user's commitment to a project.

Preliminary Analysis

To make the project request policy effective, the central computer resources manager (CCRM) must acknowledge receipt of the form. This can be a simple telephone call and brief memo explaining how the request will be reviewed. The request form initiates the preliminary analysis.

The preliminary analysis leads to the first step of defining the request or problem in terms of need. This may not be as easy as it sounds. Complaints and requests for computer systems may hide the real problem. For example, a physician who suggests that the laboratory system needs a faster printer to speed printing of daily chart reports may not understand that the delay in getting the results into the charts is that the nurse-secretaries do not begin to work until 7 a.m. The problem may be traced to physicians making their rounds at 6 a.m.

To identify the real problem to be solved, the CR staff conducts interviews, surveys users, and studies the current system. This preliminary analysis may uncover alternative solutions or show that the suggested change will result in unexpected costs, be technologically unfeasible, or be operationally unfeasible. A recommendation will be made as to whether to proceed, solve the problem another way, or recognize no feasible solution.

Users often find that enforcement of the request policy makes it easier for them to plan work schedules and focus on high priority tasks. In addition,

Figure 6-1. Computer resources project request form. Reprinted from *Managing Hospital Information Systems* by S. L. Priest, 1982, p. 99, with permission of Aspen Publication, Inc.

COMPUTER RESOURCES
PROJECT REQUEST FORM

REQUESTED BY: ______________________________

DATE REQUESTED: _____ DEPARTMENT: ______________________________

DATE NEEDED, IF CRITICAL, PLEASE EXPLAIN. ______________________________

____

PRESENT SYSTEM: ______________________________

____

PROPOSED PROJECT DESCRIPTION. STATE HOW IT MEETS AN ORGANIZATION OR DEPARTMENT STRATEGIC/OPERATIONAL OBJECTIVE: ______________________________

____

REDUCE COSTS. ANNUAL SAVINGS $_______ WHERE? ______________________________

PRODUCE ADDITIONAL INCOME. ANNUAL AMOUNT $______ HOW? ______________

IMPROVE ACCURACY AND/OR TIMELINESS OF INFORMATION. HOW? __________

REGULATORY REQUIREMENT. WHO? ______________________________

OTHER. PLEASE EXPLAIN. ______________________________

____

**************************COMPUTER RESOURCE FILL IN BELOW******************************

START DATE: ____________ ESTIMATED COMPLETION DATE: ______________________

ESTIMATED MANPOWER: ______________________________

ASSIGNED TO: ______________________________

______________________________ DATE: __________

users recognize the policy as an impartial method that acknowledges each request and ranks it in a formal priority. Chapter 8, further explains project ranking methods.

Independent User Requests

Requests that appear to affect only an individual user area, but that require purchases and process changes, should also be submitted to the CCRM. The request can then be evaluated to determine whether other areas will be affected, whether the requested purchase already exists elsewhere in the organization, or whether CR staff is needed for support. For example, a user may suggest an enhancement through a low cost microcomputer package. When it arrives, he may find that there is no documentation, that very costly training is required, that no storage space is available, or that the package is incompatible with the microcomputer being used. The CR staff might have been able to provide input into these concerns before purchase.

Feasibility Study

If the results of the inception phase of the SLC are positive, it is further refined to produce a more detailed feasibility study. The feasibility study must detail the problem and the alternatives considered and make a recommendation. The documentation of the feasibility study will include an explanation of the present system, the needs analysis and assessment (including what problems were uncovered during the study), alternative solutions considered and hidden problems, and a recommendation. If large, the problem may also require a brief financial analysis and staff needs schedule.

A Tool for Defining Needs and Solutions

The task of defining how a system functions and its various steps and processes, as well as the task of providing alternative answers and solutions, is more of an art than a science. However, there are two "tricks" that one can use to help to arrive at a system definition and solution. One technique is simply to ask what, where, why, how, who, and when questions: "What are you trying to accomplish? Where is it being done now? Who does it now? Why is it being done? How is it being done? When is it being done?" These questions, asked during the feasibility, analysis, and design phases of the SLC, allow one to focus in on the definition of the problem, process, and system.

Figure 6-2. System analysis tools for definition and alternative solutions.

As one defines a system, process, and need, ask questions for each function:

1. What?
2. Where?
3. Who?
4. Why?
5. How?
6. When?

As one tries to provide alternative solutions to a system, process, and step, ask the following:

1. Can we eliminate this?
2. Can we simplify this?
3. Can we combine this?
4. Can we change this?

A second technique, after the problem, process, and system are understood, is to provide alternative solutions by addressing each step in the process and system with the question of whether it can be eliminated, combined, simplified, or changed: "Can this step (or need) be eliminated? Can it be combined? Can it be simplified? Can it be changed?" The results of these questions are alternative solutions. Figure 6-2 summarizes the question tools, which are appropriate throughout all phases of the SLC.

The Feasibility Study Recommendation

If the recommendation is to proceed and the computer system requires major funding and staffing, the recommendation will need to be ranked by the computer resources steering committee. Chapter 8 discusses in detail how priorities for computer resource requests are addressed.

Systems Analysis

The next phase of the SLC is the systems analysis phase. In this phase, the existing procedures are detailed in more exhaustive detail than in the feasibility study. The boundaries of the computer system are defined. Data on volumes, decision points, existing files, and relationships with other computer systems are collected.

The proposed system must be defined in detail so that all can understand. The requirements of the proposed system are reviewed continually by end-users and management for feasibility and completeness. Extensive interviews with users and other concerned parties are necessary.

The results of the systems analysis are the requirements—organizational commitment, user commitment, and staff and funding needs. The systems analysis is reviewed by management to determine whether the original objectives identified in the feasibility phase are still obtainable. This report provides management an opportunity to reconsider the priority of this computer system.

System Design

The systems analysis phase of the SLC defines what is to be done, and the system design phase details how it is to be done. This is the most challenging and creative part of the SLC. There are a variety of methods available to help end-users and CR staff define the needs and requirements for a computer system. Effective methods are those that promote communication and interaction among end-users and CR staff.

Work Committee

A successful computer system must have both the support and the participation of the people who will be responsible for using and maintaining it. This is accomplished by establishing committees, herein referred to as work committees, to represent the various interests within the organization and to ensure user participation and sharing of accountability for the computer system. Members of the committee should be those having hands-on involvement in the implementation of, training for, and utilization of the system. A user manager who has no detailed understanding of the system should not be a member. A computer system may affect various areas in different ways and might therefore require more than one work committee.

The work committee can be chaired by a central CR staff member or by an end-user. The needed quality is one of being able to assign duties to the members and being able to act as a mediator and facilitator when there is a need. The chairperson must be a "make things happen" person.

Minicase 1: A Functional Work Committee

After the inception, feasibility, and analysis phases of the SLC and as part of the system design phase, the CR steering committee determined that vendor-supplied application software would be utilized. The request for proposal was sent out, and numerous vendor proposals were evaluated. One vendor was selected to provide a turnkey medical information system that included order entry and results features for nurses and physicians to request patient tests and review pending or final results. The CCRM identified a work committee to be responsible for planning, training, and implementing the system's radiology routines.

The committee membership included participants both "above" (who are in need of, or use the information) and "below" (who are responsible for feeding information up). The committee comprised a radiology supervisor, a radiologist, a dietician, a head nurse, a physician, a CR analyst, and a representative from the vendor's firm. During the first committee meeting, the committee defined its role in the system life cycle process.

The committee began by documenting present radiology patient order requests and results inquiry procedures, including the people, departments, and policies involved with the test. For example, a nurse ordering an upper GI series would need to call radiology for an appointment, notify transport that a wheelchair was needed, call dietary to hold the meal, and prepare a patient charge slip. Documentation was the responsibility of each person on the committee in his or her respective area. The system documentation as written by each member was reviewed and flow-charted by the analyst. It is at this phase that the system definition process could have resulted in expansion of the committee to include members not previously recognized as having an interest in the radiology routines.

Each committee member learned the capabilities and procedures of the radiology routines. The committee developed a plan and assigned responsibility to various members for collecting the necessary input data needs. The nursing representative was given the task of defining computer-generated nursing prep orders. By knowing the current procedures and the computer system's procedures, the committee was able to identify changes required by the vendor and by the in-house staff.

It was necessary for the committee to do pilot studies before a decision could be made on which method of data entry is best at the nursing station: keyboard, light pen, etc. This meant that the nursing member and others had to test different methods of input in addition to the committee's review of methods used at other organizations.

Once the necessary procedural changes had ben defined, the next step was to develop an installation schedule with the vendor. The schedule included both the initial system orientation sessions and ongoing in-house training programs for the nursing and ancillary departments.

The committee also provided environmental data on the present radiology order entry climate, such as the numbers of procedures per station, telephone calls to ancillary areas, duplicate orders, lost orders, etc. These parameters must be identified before system implementation to allow effective follow-up analysis, as discussed in Chapter 8.

Staff updates and procedures were prepared, with each person on the committee responsible for his or her respective area. The techniques for interaction discussed in Chapter 2 all come into play in a work committee.

Work committees should be used regardless of whether a system is being developed in-house, a turnkey package is being installed by the in-house staff or vendor, or the system is run on a computer located outside the organization. Work committees make both user and CR staffs responsible and accountable for the success of the system. Certainly the vendor must be held responsible for certain aspects of the system but, because users are the ultimate recipients of the system, they must have control over project scheduling and system acceptance specifications. Other assignments of the committee depend on the depth of the application, the degree of vendor involvement, and whether the information system affects one or more user areas.

User Groups

A unique resource can be of great assistance when implementing and selecting information systems. This resource falls under the name of "computer user groups." A computer user group is generally an organization of peers who share ideas and experiences. Participating executives have found that sharing their problems and solutions is rewarding—both professionally to the individual and financially to the institution.

Unanticipated occurrences during project definition and implementation can often affect scheduled target dates. Further, the cost and staff-hours associated with the design and implementation of a system that already exists at another organization can often be avoided. In addition, a CCRM may delay a decision to gain a better understanding of a situation and to plan for conceivable events. Meanwhile, the user can become frustrated with project delays that seem to be caused by a lack of CR staff commitment. However, the CCRM is quite aware that first-time development efforts can often be quite expensive, time-consuming, and even disastrous if not thought out very carefully. Computer user groups can aid this decision process.

A computer user group offers dialogue with one's peers. The executive can gain confidence in decisions regarding which information system to select and be able to anticipate events with an assurance that comes from actual experiences of project development.

For the organization about to embark on the development of a computer system, these meetings can provide insights and solutions to various problems and concerns. The opinions and ideas expressed by those who have attempted similar undertakings will often disclose areas that had not been previously considered. For instance, an agency preparing to implement an inventory computer system can discuss installation approaches with others who have already gone through the experience of an inventory implementation. Based on these discussions, the agency may decide that it is best to delay the printing of purchase orders until the initial system changes have been installed because the experience of others shows that procedural and personnel changes must be made over a period of time. Without firsthand inventory implementation experience, one may not have recognized this potential problem, and the installation could have been disastrous if people had to learn all of the system's features immediately.

User groups are usually organized along various lines of common interest. For instance, the Cooperative Health-Care User Group (CHUG) and Electronic Computing Health Oriented (ECHO) are both vocation- and vendor-oriented. The members have an interest in the health-care field, and all use the same hardware vendor. Organizations using the same software vendor likewise have user groups. Other groups have the common interest of being located in the same area, such as the New England Computer User Group (NECUG). A user group whose members all program in the same language is the MUMPS Users Group. The Data Processing Management Association (DPMA) is a less specialized association open to all persons interested in data processing regardless of vocation, vendor, or location. The frequency of association meetings can vary from monthly to annually.

Attendance at a user group meeting presents an excellent opportunity for exchanging ideas with vendors and evaluating various vendor offerings through discussions and seminars presented by users and vendors. This exchange can result in improved utilization of CRs through an awareness of vendor offerings. Discussions with vendors can include system operating techniques, dissatisfaction with vendor services, and upcoming vendor announcements. The group meetings provide an opportunity to attend state-of-the-art educational sessions in software, hardware, management, and other topics necessary for the continued professional development of both the user and the CR staffs.

A vendor can financially support a group, or a group can be self-supporting through member dues and meeting registration fees. There are various publications such as Data*mation* and *Computerworld*, which announce meeting dates, mailing addresses, and brief descriptions for nearly all user groups. Also, vendors usually publish announcements of their own user group meetings.

While attending user group meetings, one establishes peer contacts that are invaluable when seeking reference checks on potential employees. References from user group contacts can provide frank and candid responses that can give one confidence when making a hiring decision. In addition, some user groups have newsletters to announce position openings.

When an organization is evaluating a vendor, attendance at a vendor-oriented meeting can provide valuable information from current users on that vendor's ability to meet one's computer resource needs. In addition, the degree of user satisfaction with the vendor's services usually becomes obvious with the general tone of a user meeting.

Sometimes, a visit to a vendor-recommended organization may not present a true picture of their satisfaction with the vendor if the visitor is not known to the organization being visited. Previous contact with the users at a user group meeting can result in valuable insights into vendor deficiencies that may not be gained during a vendor-arranged site visit.

A user group may make application software available to members at a fraction of the development cost and save an organization thousands of dollars in project costs. These potential cost savings can justify attendance at a group meeting. During evaluation of user- and vendor-developed software applications, the comments from one's peers will provide a means of judging the adequacy of the software and its documentation.

User groups usually publish a membership catalog, which can be used as a routine resource in identifying organizations of similar size and hardware that have developed application packages. An executive trying to select a microbiology system can use the catalog to identify organizations that have already developed and implemented the application. A simple telephone call or letter to that agency can then reveal whether the listed package should be further considered.

Membership in a user group may also assure one of extensive vendor service through a user committee providing a liaison between members and vendors for seemingly unsolvable problems. For instance, if an organization is having hardware or software delivery problems, the committee may be able to assist in circumventing the often time-consuming task of waiting for follow-through on the problem.

There are times when one will question a vendor's policy or stance on a subject. The salesperson's response may be, "that's the way it is!" The same question presented to a corporate officer in front of a user group meeting may result in a different response and further comments from the membership. Frequently, vendor officers attend user meetings and are available for formal and informal discussions. Often, an informal, semisocial, off-the-cuff conversation with a corporate officer can pay enormous dividends.

Some user groups have established a committee that maintains an amicable software and hardware dialogue between vendor and user. These committees encourage user recommendations and suggestions and, after committee agreement, forward a recommendation to the vendor for implementation. Usually, a recommendation from a committee that represents many users will carry more weight with the vendor than the request of one user.

Minicase 2: A User Group Meeting

The following account of an actual situation might best serve to summarize the effectiveness of a user group. An unseasoned CCRM was given the responsibility of staffing a CR department and recommending computer system implementation priorities. The organization had been purchasing computer services from a shared vendor and wanted its own CR staff. The CCRM was to staff the department, recommend to the CRs steering committee the sequence and the priorities of each application that was to be converted from the shared vendor, and determine whether the application software should be purchased or developed in-house. In addition, the organization's steering committee had limited CR experience, which meant that the inexperienced CCRM was without an in-house CR peer.

In addition to the CCRM's inexperience, the software vendor was complicating the situation by directly contacting steering committee members and promising exaggerated implementation schedules and grandiose packages. The CCRM decided to attend a computer user group meeting that had the common interest of health care and the software vendor.

The CCRM, a gregarious person, did not hesitate to inform the group of his rather limited background and asked for suggestions and opinions. Through the cooperation of the members, the CCRM was able to identify areas of concern that had to be addressed to accomplish the monumental task. Formal and informal discussions with people who had faced similar situations revealed varied experiences. Problems such as staffing needs were discussed and, after hearing various opinions, the CCRM was able to judge what was best for his organization. When the question of which application to implement was asked, it was learned that each package required its own implementation plan as well as various degrees of implementation experience. Thus, the sequence of implementation could be important, allowing one to acquire more in-house experience as well as compatible interfaces between packages.

The CCRM was able to document and justify to the committee a recommended implementation schedule and an organizational structure for CR staffing. The experiences of user group members were an invaluable resource to the rapidly maturing CCRM.

Utilizing the computer to its fullest potential calls for vast amounts of learning and experience. CR knowledge can certainly be gained through trial and error—a long, costly, and inefficient process. A user group can be used to help minimize this expenditure of time and money by making available the hard-won skill, knowledge, and experience of other member professionals.

System Development

The purpose of the system development phase of the SLC is to build a system that meets the requirements specified in the previous phases. The system may be purchased, or it may be developed in-house. New procedures may be designed so that people will know how to use the system. The use of a request for proposal (RFP) and the needs assessment process discussed in Chapter 4 is an essential part of the system development phase of the SLC.

User Interaction

The necessity of user interaction is a must for a successful information system implementation. All interested parties must be contacted when planning the implementation strategy. The degree of interaction of the user is discussed in this chapter and is further detailed in Chapter 3.

Monitoring Progress

A Gantt chart, critical path chart, and other scheduling techniques can be used to provide visual awareness of the progress of the computer system. All parties concerned with the computer system should be aware of its status through memos and work committee meetings and reports.

Understanding Needs

It is often difficult to comprehend fully a system's actual requirements or perceive the full system's effect on the end-user and user area operation. To meet this need, the CR analyst will play a vital role as he or she works with the user to provide insight and definition of what is needed from the system.

There are various ways to provide the user with an understanding of how the system will be implemented and how the system will operate once it is installed. The analyst can provide sample reports, screen layouts, visual display charts, and flow charts for the user's comment and approval. For instance, a physician who has requested an on-line statistical summary from the patient database may not be sure of how the summary will be used or how it should be printed. As the use of the summary plays a major part in the determination of the system's reporting capabilities, the analyst can ask appropriate questions and prepare sufficient documents so that both the user and the analyst feel comfortable with what is needed and why.

Some CR managers require the user to sign off on system design and development specifications. The user's signature is supposed to ensure an understanding of and commitment to the project. However, a signature should not mandate system features that become recognized as unacceptable during implementation. Holding a user to a signature as approval of a system that is not usable is not the policy of a user-oriented CR staff. Thus, obtaining user sign-off approval is one method of ensuring a certain degree of user interaction and commitment, but the CR management must be aware of the reality that signatures may not be binding.

Structured Development and Programming Tools

CCRMs are continually confronted with new and challenging developments to improve the systems development and programming phases of the SLC. Structured walk-throughs, top-down modular design, database management systems, and structured programming techniques are but a few of the tools available to increase productivity (Amadio 1989).

Computer-aided software engineering (CASE) tools can be used to automate such system development tasks as program coding and documentation management. CASE tools support the more creative tasks of problem analysis, system design, and project management. These tools can also be used to integrate standalone products into a comprehensive environment that provides automated support for the entire SLC.

Modern software development often utilizes fourth-generation languages (4GL). Such languages used in conjunction with database management systems provide the capabilities to aid both users and programmers with screen formats, report writers, and nonprocedural programming.

Computer systems are designed upon requirements that the user believes to be realistic at the outset of the SLC. However, these initial requirements can frequently change as the user begins to see each requirement in an operational mode. Programming changes made to conform to these new requirements often cause unforeseen problems and delay the implementation schedule. In addition, the design of a program may not allow excessive coding changes. For instance, a system designed to accept only data in a particular format may have to be changed to accept another format. If, in the original coding structure, there was no consideration of additional data formats, then the recoding may take nearly as long as the original development time. Problems such as this occur frequently and are a major concern during program development.

The programming phase of the SLC cannot begin until after the system design phase is complete. The design must include output needs and reporting, input data specifications, user control procedures, and responsibilities. If programming begins before definition of the computer system specifications, major problems of systems design and software development arise. Systems and programs may not meet user requirements, and applications may not be produced on time. Applications may cost considerably more than was estimated. Programs may contain errors, and systems and programs may be difficult to change to meet new user requirements.

One may avoid these pitfalls through structured techniques for program definitions, procedures, controls, and documentation. There are many excellent references on structured systems and programming techniques for software development (Minch et al. 1982). A few of these structured techniques will now be discussed.

One tool of systems analysis that can be quite useful is Structured English. This is a specification language that is restricted to using a limited English vocabulary and syntax to describe the system's policies and logic. With Structured English, an analyst is able to involve the end-user in the logical workings of a system and program. Structured English is also a good tool for documentation and is very good for promoting interaction between users and analysts.

Another technique can be the development of a prototype minisystem for user testing and operation. This method requires that the analyst and user both address their attention to the usage of a model system. The user and CR staff have their own areas of expertise and their own vocabularies, and the communication problems that arise between user and analyst concerning systems definitions, features, and usage can be quickly identified with the minisystem approach. The analyst and user attempt to establish the fundamental requirements of the system, and then a model is programmed on the computer. This creates a minisystem, which can be easily changed to conform to user requirements. The system is essentially built and tested in serial stages, beginning with simple features and growing from there. The system is then tested for acceptability by the user under trial conditions at each stage. When the minisystem finally meets the user specifications for a stage, the system is then further developed until it eventually becomes a large scale production application.

Another structured technique designed to improve systems analysis and programmer performance, as well as user interaction and understanding of the computer system, is the structured walk-through. This is a review process where members of the CR programming staff provide review for the user and analyst. During the structured walk-through, a person on the programming team explains the system's development process, and the members critique the presentation. Meetings can occur throughout all phases of the development process, including systems definitions, programming, documentation, logic, and final testing. The walk-through not only improves the quality of the computer system, but enhances the professional development of those being reviewed via the learning experience of constructive criticism.

Structured techniques are simply tools to enhance the systems and programming process. Even with these tools, it is difficult for a user to anticipate all of the potential benefits and needs of a new or enhanced computer system. Each organization must have CR procedures and policies to determine the design of the computer system.

It is very important to require that all programming changes be tested before implementation. A small, seemingly meaningless change can have a significant effect on a computer system if not handled properly. Program errors can usually be eliminated by operating the complete system in a test mode before installation. Changes made when the system is live are strongly discouraged but, if absolutely necessary, must be very closely monitored. Whether a program change is made in-house or by a vendor, the end-user should always test its accuracy before and after the change is "brought live."

Quality Documentation

In-house and vendor documentation of the system and programs is essential. This documentation must be mandated by CR policy. Documentation standards should include the other programs and systems with which the programs interface, flow charts, program specifications, record layouts, and definitions of all terms used. Backup and recovery procedures should also be documented. The quality of the computer system is directly proportional to the amount of documentation provided.

On-line programming development software can assist in real-time documentation while the program is being prepared. Documentation is as essential as the actual programs and, although sometimes seeming questionable, may someday be the only thing standing between the organization and disaster. Documentation should be reviewed and approved by the person responsible for the computer system.

End-user Development

It would be safe to say that the vast majority of user areas will never program their microcomputer systems. They will purchase vendor-provided microcomputer software such as integrated packages that provide word processing, spreadsheet, graphics, downloading, and telecommunications. The system development phase of the SLC recognizes that the majority of users will use vendor-provided software and 4GLS rather than going through a structured programming process.

In-house Development versus Vendor Software

A decision to develop application software in-house, acquire software from vendors for in-house modification, or acquire totally vendor-supported software depends on the existence and sophistication of the software available and the expertise of the CR and user staffs. Organizations faced with a choice of in-house or vendor-provided software should most often select the vendor-provided software. Vendor software is justified because in-house software development usually costs many times that of acquiring a vendor's product. Vendor development costs can be spread out among many customers, whereas in-house development costs are borne by a single organization. In addition, the difficulty of procuring the time and CR staff necessary to design and develop in-house software may automatically prohibit it.

An implementation deadline for an application may determine that it be acquired from an outside source. An organization faced with a mandatory implementation date, such as one that has been told that its time-sharing payroll vendor is going out of business within three months, will have to acquire an outside payroll package immediately to avoid interrupting normal operation.

The extensive time and cost of in-house development for an already existing application usually does not justify the trials and tribulations of system definition, programming, and debugging. Furthermore, a more complicated and unique application, such as a financial budgeting and simulation system, requires esoteric knowledge and insight, such as continual monitoring of legislative mandates and necessitates dedicating extensive CR staff with the risk of never completing the application.

An organization would never want to develop software for a comprehensive laboratory system. The years have seen many software vendors come and go from laboratory development, as the software is very complicated and takes years to shape and debug. The required costs, staff, and time prohibit most organizations from even thinking about such development.

If an application is available, but does not fit the exact requirements and needs of the user, one may decide to purchase the general package and then modify it in-house or with outside contract vendors so that it will fit the user's specific situation and need. In this case, the extent and type of modifications necessary to the general package must be carefully weighed because extensive changes can result in a commitment of the CR staff comparable to that required for in-house development. A user change in a vendor program may violate the vendor's maintenance agreement, and the vendor may not support the user if the application does not work.

Most vendors shy away from supporting a user-modified package because the vendor staff essentially needs to start from the beginning to learn how the modification has affected the package. Furthermore, the package may interface with other applications, and extensive time may be necessary simply to understand where changes differ from the standard package and the effect on other packages caused by the modifications. Thus, most users will pay the vendor to provide this level of customization and to maintain coverage by the vendor on other applications. Restrictions (such as funding) may limit in-house staff size, making it highly risky to modify vendor applications.

Vendors may not take the user's, or even the user-purchased, custom programs into consideration when introducing new application features. Thus, the user may find that the new features of an application are not compatible with existing programs.

Another consideration when deciding the source of a software system is the use of contract programmers to supplement staff development. Contract programmers can often eliminate the need for hiring additional permanent staff when a development effort is either temporary or just behind schedule. When selecting this alternative, one must be sure that the service provided by the contract programmer is clearly defined and that the programmer is familiar with the application. Without clear program instructions and an understanding of the application, the time and effort to educate outside assistance may negate potential savings. In some cases, contract programmers may be even more costly and may cause in-house staff disruptions. In addition, the type of written program documentation that the contract programmer provides should be carefully reviewed, as inadequate documentation can be a source of frustration for the in-house staff who later may assume the maintenance of these programs.

There are various sources from which to acquire proven software packages. One common source is the many hardware vendors who have a variety of application packages either developed by their own staff or purchased from their customers. Another source is software brokers' market packages that have been developed by individual software houses, but the programming quality and documentation should be reviewed carefully to ensure completeness and accuracy. A third source is a user group, as discussed previously in this chapter. User groups traditionally offer self-developed software for minimal costs. However, there may be minimal systems and programming support to the packages, and documentation should bc carefully reviewed for its existence, completeness, and currency.

Users should ensure that any procedural and operational changes necessary because of package requirements will meet the end-user's needs. Using the RFP and needs definition process of the systems development phase of the SLC will minimize end-user disruption and adversity.

Training, Conversion, and Installation

Training

Training is essential for smooth conversion and installation. Users develop materials and conduct training sessions. The work committee must oversee the training schedules and work closely with the user computer resource manager (UCRM) to provide any needed resources.

Make Changes before Installing the Computer System

If possible, one should implement procedural and policy changes before the installation of the computer system. If workflow changes are made before equipment installation or before reports and screens are generated, implementation will be less traumatic. Hardware and software installations concurrent with procedure changes can often mask the cause of an implementation problem. Problems associated with procedures can be identified more easily than problems of hardware and software. Therefore, the transition to a new system is easier to control if the changes are phased into a user's normal operations and procedures. Programming changes often must be made to conform with end-user policy. These policy changes can be quickly identified before programming begins.

An example of changes that can be made before conversion involves a radiology order system. Because most computer systems require the user to input a procedure name using a specific mnemonic code, it is possible to require users to begin using specific mnemonics when placing orders on paper, even before the computer arrives. For example, a chest X-ray would be ordered on the form as "CXT." Thus, all users would feel comfortable with the order nomenclature before the computer is installed.

Another example is an emergency department system to monitor consumer products responsible for accidents. The first phase of this new computer system might be to have the nurses and admitting clerks enter into the patient record the individual product mnemonics that may have caused the accident. The second phase of implementation would then involve the actual computer system and using the visual display unit (VDU) to capture the data. In this approach, the user did not have to learn two procedures at once, but gradually phased in each change.

Another example might be an agency about to install a computer system to analyze its client patients. It is known that all visiting nurses will be required to fill out a data collection form for each patient seen. The form can be designed and used before the computer system is installed. Thus, the person who will complete the form can use a variety of forms to test the ease of transcribing the appropriate input data. Furthermore, the data collected as part of the test can also be used to test the programs. Changes required of a user should be scheduled to ease user acceptance.

Time to Adjust

Vendor software contracts will usually insist on an orientation period of three to four months before additional program changes are considered. Many of the required procedures that accompany a new system demand an adjustment period before the full effect of the system can be evaluated. A period of time is necessary before the user accepts the system as routine. During this adjustment period, there should be a minimal number of programming changes (except for bugs!) until the system has been fully installed. Once the routines of the system and procedures are understood, the user can discuss and request changes through the Request Form in Figure 6-1.

Data Protection, Security, Confidentiality, and Computer Viruses

Reliance on computer resources for quality patient care, decision-making, and financial management mandates three basic concerns when using computers: (1) physical security for databases, software, and hardware; (2) systems security for data and program integrity; and (3) data confidentiality to restrict access to those with a need to know.

One hundred percent security and confidentiality for a computer system cannot be guaranteed (Bruce 1984, Minard 1987). However, many problems of security and confidentiality can be prevented, anticipated, and minimized by both the CR and the user staffs through planning, policies, audits, and procedures.

The incidence of reported computer crime has increased with the awareness of "computer viruses." Computer viruses are programs that systematically destroy other programs and generally disrupt user confidence in computer resources. Analogous to a biological virus, a computer virus is planted in the computer and then makes the copies of itself on data storage devices and in microcomputers in the network, destroying some or all of the data and programs or consuming space at rates that essentially use up all available storage. There are now several generations of computer-literate people and with that literacy has come increased exposure to potential loss.

A physical security plan requires not only policies for the prevention of harm to hardware, software, supplies, and databases, but also procedures that will adequately replace or substitute items if destruction does occur. Physical harm can come to a facility through acts of nature, vandalism, or (the most common occurrence) accidents and mistakes caused by its own employees. One can prevent many of these occurrences through personnel policies, training, and restricting access to computer facilities and terminals (Clarke and Prins 1986). The appendix details a scenario of a physician group practice that learned about data protection the hard way.

An organization should always have a tested disaster plan that provides for off-site operation in case of facility destruction or loss of access (as could occur during an employee strike). This plan can include a written agreement with the off-site facility to operate in a batch mode or possibly on-line time-sharing modes (although the chances of on-line backup are usually slim). This backup site should be periodically used to run the software and databases to ensure compatibility of operations. For on-line processing, this backup site is usually more difficult to arrange and use because the site will itself be operating on-line. Also, the required communication hardware may make it difficult to locate a perfectly compatible site. Also, the task of changeover may make off-site on-line backup difficult.

Another backup site alternative is a duplicate facility, usually known as a shell, where another off-site building is prepared and maintained in case of destruction to the main facility. Most organizations today do not have such an arrangement because of its obvious cost, but instead have a disaster plan that includes manual procedures that will substitute for the on-line systems in case of an emergency. The use of manual procedures for more than a few weeks is questionable because it would be very difficult to maintain order for an extended period.

Another method of off-site backup is dependence on the hardware vendor for equipment. Vendor policies should be reviewed to determine whether hardware replacement after a disaster can be guaranteed within a certain number of days. However, depending on the complexity of one's hardware configuration, a 100% compatibility with hardware and communication needs may be difficult to achieve.

Systems and software security techniques and procedures for data and programming integrity are numerous. The purpose is to minimize the amount of "polluted" data entering databases, prevent the loss of data, and provide audit trails for the identification of system programming problems. People and equipment are subject to failures and errors, such as power shortages, hardware malfunctions, and program logic problems, and programs and data must be capable of being recovered if a system suddenly halts.

There are many system techniques for recovery. For instance, if an online patient registration system that continually updates patient databases throughout the day suddenly comes to a halt, the structure of the programs should be such that the system is capable of restarting with minimal data loss. This may mean continually logging transactions to duplicate magnetized disk or tape databases. Routine backup procedures protect against data loss when hardware and software fail. The choicc of which backup procedure to use depends on the cost and time necessary if the data and programs must be recovered. An office using a microcomputer may save their data onto disks or magnetic tape once a day.

An installation with critical applications that will not tolerate even minimal system failure and downtime will require duplicate hardware, such as fault-tolerant or duplication computers that could handle the work of the other units, albeit in a degraded mode, until the computer is repaired. The high costs of uninterrupted power supplies are necessary for those organizations that must have the computers available 24 hours a day. On-line systems should have backup requirements that are capable of data and program recovery and restart with no loss of stored data.

Application software and data must be duplicated and secured off-site. This protects against environmental disasters causing a loss of valuable and irreplaceable data. Up-to-date copies of all databases and documentation should also be kept off-site. These backup media should routinely be reviewed to make sure that they are current and should also periodically be tested at the backup site to ensure compatibility with the site's hardware and software.

There are many other security features to protect and recover programs and databases. These are usually given as checklists, as noted in many of the suggested readings at the end of this chapter.

Users are very much concerned with the confidentiality of their databases. As the number of computer-sorted databases increases, all users must be assured that their databases are protected from illegal access and theft. Because of this, many user areas still maintain manual databases and files in order to have control over certain confidential data. These files can contain data not stored in the computer, but there are a variety of methods to provide users with confidentiality of computer-stored data.

One method is to require a computer password for authorized users. When the person using an access terminal is properly identified, such as through identification codes, names, and even handprints, the authorized users file can be further interrogated to determine what information the person is authorized to access and whether the person is further permitted to insert and alter existing data. The computer can maintain a log of each person accessing the database and the nature of his or her inquiry. Users and auditors can periodically review who has been accessing the database. With the use of this method, computer databases are often more private and secure than manual record-keeping files. Whereas manual files can be searched and updated without any visible audit trail, a computer log lists all users of the file.

The wide usage of telecommunications today has made computer access even more prominent. It takes only a modem, a telephone number, and knowledge of access codes to dial into a database. Features such as dial-back software can prevent unauthorized access into a database.

Federal and state legislation on patient and employee privacy, confidentiality, and data accuracy must continually be reviewed by both the user and the CR management. The National Commission on Confidentiality of Health Records is a group working to create confidentiality standards and frequently publishes on the subject.

In general, as you make it more difficult for unauthorized users to gain access, it gets more difficult for authorized users, too. It can be very frustrating for a user who has to type three passwords to gain access. If people get frustrated, they find ways around the security, thus rendering it useless. Users and organizations must weigh their security needs against efficiency needs and seek a prudent balance between the two; they should not implement so many security devices and procedures that the CR become unusable, but neither should they leave valuable and confidential data unprotected.

Another subject of concern for the user and the CR staff is the potential destruction and harm that can come through user and CR staff negligence and fraud. Fraud is one concern that both the user and the CR management find very difficult to handle and monitor. If a person wants to cheat the system, or even destroy it, he or she most likely can find a way. Policies for the hiring and termination of employees can be used to address this problem. These include extensive reference checks before hiring an employee and immediate termination of employees who give notice. Periodic job rotation of computer operators, programmers, and user terminal operators should be required. Vacations should be mandated for these same people.

One area that requires close scrutiny is the design and physical layout of the computer facility. For this purpose, CR managers usually bring in computer environmental experts for consultation. Items such as a locked computer area and a sign-in/sign-out book offer protection for the facility.

This text will not address the various methods of legal protection for software. Readers may consult the suggested readings for a thorough explanation of software patent, copyright, and trade secret laws.

In summary, an organization is faced with a pressing need to build adequate safeguards into all computer systems. This need can be met only through continual monitoring and enhancements of security and confidentiality plans, procedures, and policies. Computer resources can be protected from loss or unauthorized access by:

- Employees should be screened effectively.
- Users should not be given carte blanche access to data. There must be prescribed levels of access, with the user's level of access based on the need to know.
- Data must be duplicated routinely and stored off-site at a restricted facility.
- Users must be educated as to the need for security and data protection. Signed password forms must be used.
- Users must not leave their computers unattended or give their passwords to another user. Passwords must not be posted on walls or written as part of user manuals.
- Double sign-on procedures will not allow a user access to data without another user signing on simultaneously.
- Software programs can be run to check for computer viruses.
- The organization can purchase hardware such as callback modems.
- Users should not be allowed to bring developed software from or to home.

- Smart cards and encryption devices can be used to send data between computers and to identify authorized users.
- Computer-maintained user logs can monitor the usage of applications, VDTs, and data.
- Voice, fingerprint, or retina can be used for positive identification.
- Outside access to computers can be monitored using printers connected to the computer line to list all data input and output from the computer.
- Computer usage areas can be designed for maximal security.
- Unauthorized users should be terminated and prosecuted.
- A comprehensive CR security policy must be developed on an ongoing basis.
- Security considerations must be addressed when new hardware and software are purchased.
- User jobs should be rotated.
- Frequent changing of passwords is helpful.
- Passwords should not be simple to guess. One-character passwords and other obvious ones such as names and birthdates should be discouraged. A password checker program can be used to avoid obvious and easily guessed passwords.
- At least annual testing of on-site and off-site computer disaster plans should be done.
- Up-to-date documentation should be maintained, with at least an annual sign-off by users and CR staffs certifying that manuals are current and understood.
- There should be an annual check-off list audit of computer resources for the listed concerns, such as the current password list (i.e., no terminated employees with active passwords, follow-up on computer data rejects, and other CR policies and guidelines).

Conversion Techniques

Converting from one information system to another, whether manual or automated, involves cooperation and mutual planning to minimize user disruption and errors. Planning includes education and training of the user staff before conversion. The conversion of certain systems, such as order entry, has organization-wide implications and requires full cooperation of administration, finance, nursing, medical staff, and ancillary staff. Other systems, such as payroll, have an organization-wide financial impact, and there may be little room for conversion error.

During the selection and planning stages, the user and CR staff will have an opportunity to judge the adequacy of user procedures, as well as the ability of personnel to adjust to the system and to changes in procedures. Users are then prepared for their expected role in the conversion. Users must fully understand their role in the conversion and be aware of problems that can occur if the conversion is not made properly. There are many examples of less than successful computer system installations due to users not being properly prepared for their role in the conversion and maintenance process.

Comparison Testing. One effective technique for the conversion of information systems is to operate parallel current and future systems. This means running both the new and the old systems side by side and comparing the results. The user will compare the output of both systems to ensure compatibility. The work effort can often be reduced if the same input data are adaptable to both systems, eliminating the preparation of redundant data.

Minicase 3: A Parallel Scheduling Test

To ensure the accuracy of a new nurse scheduling system, the users maintained parallel manual and real-time systems. The nursing supervisor continued to prepare by hand the daily scheduling report using completed input forms from each nursing station. The supervisor used the same forms for input into the computer system. This allowed the supervisor to determine whether the calculations and reporting features of both the manual and the automated systems were compatible. Furthermore, this parallel method allowed the supervisor to learn the new system through reconciling system differences between the manual and automated systems. This reconciliation process demonstrated to the supervisor that the manual report had frequent calculation errors and took three weeks longer to prepare than the automated report. Thus, the new system was accepted with enthusiasm by the supervisor. The parallel conversion also gave the supervisor an understanding of the inner workings of the scheduling system, which resulted in the supervisor identifying and correcting procedural problems.

A parallel test can cover various time periods and should verify as many system features as is reasonable. For instance, an organization converting to a new payroll system may schedule the parallel when the weekly, monthly, quarterly, and end-of-the-year periods are concurrent, thereby maximizing the number of system features that can be checked within a limited parallel schedule.

Parallels can often reveal existing deficiencies in current systems. A pharmacy was converting its formulary to a new system. It printed a hard copy of the old formulary and, using a magnetic tape, converted the file to the new system and printed a supposedly duplicate hard copy. A comparison of the old and new reports revealed additional formularly items in the new system. An investigation located an error in the original system's program that was uncovered only when the original was compared with the new system.

The importance of balancing costs with realistic time schedules for conversion must be considered. Excessive conversion costs can be caused by maintaining two systems, as well as by overtime hours necessary to handle the increased workload. Frequently, these unwanted costs may be used to rationalize an overly optimistic conversion schedule. The results can be disastrous. For example, a conversion took place in an organization that desired to transfer the shared-service accounts-receivable system to an in-house system within a month. No time was planned for parallel testing of the new system, and the result was a rush conversion with many undetected errors that prevented the organization from printing accounts-receivable statements for nearly four months. This situation could have been prevented by developing a realistic conversion schedule that weighed the cost of a potential disaster against the cost and practicality of parallel testing.

Live and Test Programs. Duplicate sets of application programs, one for the live system and the other for testing, can be used in a real-time environment. When a feature has been proven acceptable to the user on the test program, it can then be put into the live system. The test system uses data made up by the user.

One method for teaching a user to operate and test real-time systems is to create test master files for user training. For instance, nurses can learn to order patient tests by accessing a fictitious patient and then ordering tests as if the patient were in-house. The system will simulate the actual ordering functions and perform all console lead-throughs without actually updating files. This method can also be used for ongoing in-house training for new employees.

The paralleling methods are a valuable quality control technique to minimize live system errors and also obtain user acceptance and verification of system functions. However, parallels may cause increased workloads for the user, and the length and extensiveness of a parallel may need to be curtailed.

Pilot Testing. The pilot method of testing minimizes risk by assigning a small group of users to convert directly to the new system. If the new system fails, the damage is minimal because only a small part of the user area or organization is affected. An advantage of pilot testing is that the pilot group can later serve as trainers for the new group. The following is a case in point.

A CR department and a user department were skeptical of the usefulness of computer-output-microfiche (COM) for a business office, yet both were faced with voluminous generation of paper. It was decided to do a pilot study using office volunteers to test a COM system. Each volunteer was asked to use one of four COM viewers for a week, and then the viewers were rotated. The volunteers were asked for ideas and suggestions. The testing period had served as the training period as well as convincing the business office that the new system was needed. The cost savings predicted at the beginning of the trial period were exceeded by nearly 100%. Unexpected benefits, such as reduction in turnaround time and document storage space, were also realized.

Direct Testing. The direct method of testing is the most dangerous because the organization switches immediately from the old to the new system. If the new system fails, it could hurt the entire organization but, if it succeeds, the cost of the conversion is minimal. The direct method can be used if demonstration of the new system can prove that the current system is inefficient. For this method to be effective, the people who participate in the conversion must see for themselves the need for the new system.

An example of direct testing is when the existing system has not been kept current. Manual inventory systems maintain inventory stock levels on index cards. The updating of these cards usually is not timely and frequently is incomplete. A parallel conversion between a manual system and an on-line inventory system may be frustrating when trying to reconcile differences caused by human tardiness and poor stock control. In addition, computer systems may reveal deficiencies in a manual system, as when a stock clerk can conceal with an eraser stock level differences between the card and the shelf inventory levels. A computerized inventory system will not allow this concealment to be made so easily. When converting an entirely new system where no parallel is possible, the users can provide sample data and be responsible for ensuring calculation accuracy by reconciling the system's output.

Phased Testing. With the phased method of testing, the new system is gradually phased in by introducing portions of the overall system over time. It takes longer than most other methods, but is less risky than direct testing. For example, a laboratory system might be phased in over a year, starting with chemistry, then converting bacteriology, and then the other sections.

In summary, conversion techniques may involve:

- Comparison test—i.e., parallel testing
- Live and test routines and databases
- Pilot testing
- Direct testing
- Phased testing

Operations—The Ongoing Computer System

Maintenance

After the problems of installation are resolved, the organization has adjusted to the new system on a routine basis. However, this does not mean that the system remains unchanged; there is a constant need for maintenance and enhancements. Maintenance is required because programs inevitably have errors that must be corrected. Because of the newness of the system, users and CR staff may not have communicated accurately, so that certain aspects of the system must be modified as operational experience is gained. The system life cycle begins again as the project request form is used to convey deficiencies and possible enhancements to the computer system.

Controls

Computer system controls must be easy to use while maintaining vigilance over the system's integrity. Through proper user and organizational controls, a problem can be quickly identified and then solved before the problem causes wrong decisions or financial hardships. Proper controls save time and money and promote confidence in computer resources.

The CCRM and UCRM cannot continually watch over the installed computer system, so there must be policies and procedures to ensure the detection and handling of incorrect input, the reasonableness of output reporting, and the proper maintenance of the system's database files.

An example of user controls is the operating room system using controls to ensure the correct processing of operating room data. The operative procedure log is used to update the computer for all surgical patients on a daily basis. The operating room secretary maintains a daily count of operations that should balance the computer-supplied totals. Upon entry of each data element, the computer identifies data errors. At the end of the month, the computer provides additional monthly counts to balance with the manually maintained count. It also identifies all data errors. This control technique is simple, yet effective, and ensures correct statistics that can be used to make major decisions about operating room scheduling and staffing.

The use of real-time systems makes control a different challenge than with paperwork. Real-time systems can require VDT security codes, access restrictions, and time of day access. For instance, nursing may only access patients on the same floor as the terminal. Further, only people with a certain security code can enter test requests. Other systems can restrict access to selected functions during certain hours of the day. For instance, if it is known that there is no physical therapy (PT) activity after 5 p.m., the system can restrict access to PT files after 5 p.m.

Controls can be built into a systems program to examine output reasonableness. For instance, a laboratory system may have normal range checks on test results to assist in quality control. If a test result falls outside the normal range, the computer will flag it for review by the user manager.

Routine review of transaction reports should be sent to each area's UCRM. These reports represent all transactions that have gone through the user areas, the files accessed and updated, the persons using the VDTs, and the exact time and duration of VDT usage. These reports can be audited for unusual activity (such as unauthorized access of files, excessive attempts at VDT access with the wrong password, and excessive errors), which may indicate that additional training or security is necessary.

Programming the computer to edit data being entered while also maintaining computer error reports can be an excellent management control. These error reports can be reviewed by user managers to identify the type of errors and the people who are making them.

A medical records department was having a problem of patients being issued duplicate medical record numbers. Investigation showed that the problem was caused by admitting clerks overriding a four-step identification procedure, resulting in the issuing of new medical record numbers before a patient was thoroughly screened for an existing number. Using the computer to force the mandatory four-step process was an obvious solution, but this would have caused unacceptable time delays because many patients, such as newborns, did not have to go through the four-step process. The solution was having the computer generate an audit report that identified the registration clerk and the step that was used to issue the number. Now the admitting supervisor can quickly identify the clerks who do not follow the required registration procedure.

Systems that go unwatched can often be expensive to correct. An example is a home health agency that did not closely monitor its accounts-receivable database. At the end of the month, it was determined by the internal auditor that the computer monthly reports differed from the expected by more than $60,000. It was discovered that a clerk had mistakenly used the wrong disk to run a daily update, and the error was not detected until three weeks later. Consequently, the office has instituted controls that now compare computer daily file totals to month-to-date computer-generated totals. In addition, at the end of the month, reports are further reconciled against external control before delivery.

Proper updating and maintenance of documentation is a vital control to ensure that all systems and program enhancements are available. Such controls may be as simple as requiring yearly review and a supervisor's signature on all documentation manuals. If turnover in a user area occurs and a manual has not been kept updated, the system may gradually become ineffective and even be abandoned. Documentation ensures that the painstaking efforts of all involved will be permanent and will transcend changes in the user area.

An accounting department did an internal audit of its own area, which showed many manual record-keeping systems that duplicated existing, but unused, computer-maintained databases as well as report features. As employee turnover in the department occurred, many of the system's reporting features were not explained to the new staff. Because the end-user manual was also not maintained, it was never used in employee training and, in a four-year period, more than 25% of the system's features had been forgotten.

The preparation of journal articles can also be a form of control. An article describing the use of a computer system published in a national journal both documents the system benefits and demonstrates the organization's successful system. The recognition that the facility receives from publishing will encourage the user department to maintain the system at its optimal level as well as continue to improve it. Visits by other interested organizations further encourage documentation of the system. Site visits require end-users to continue to learn the system, and an additional benefit is what one usually learns from the visitor. One must know the system to explain it to others, and the questions of others encourage new insights.

The sharing of software and procedures among organizations maintains and enhances programs as well as their accompanying documentation. When one shares a system, the receiver new to the system must have proper user, system, and programming documentation. Errors in the software coding and documentation found by the recipient can be brought to the attention of the giver, thus further debugging the system and assuring the system's integrity.

This section has described many control procedures that can be applied to a computer system. These techniques are necessary whether a user area maintains its own system, has access to a CR staff, or receives services from outside vendors. An organization that continually reviews its systems and practices interaction techniques will solve problems as they occur and promote confidence and pride in computer resources.

Postimplementation Studies

Over the course of a long project, an expected benefit may be forgotten or put aside. A follow-up study made at three to six months after installation will show whether the system features are being used and, if not, why. Follow-up studies are an important phase of the SLC. They are discussed in detail in Chapter 8.

Systems Evaluation and Follow-up

The postimplementation phase of the systems life cycle is often considered the final phase of the project. In reality, however, no project is ever really complete. There is continual need to evaluate the ongoing costs of a project and the system's ability to change and meet the needs of the user.

Cost Evaluation

Comparing year-by-year costs of computer resources for an organization or specialty is one way to evaluate the return on the organization's CR investment. For example, an organization can review industry statistics for costs in a comparable organization and then determine whether its own costs are in line with industry standards. A 250-bed hospital can compare its CR-adjusted patient day cost with published standards and make a determination of whether its own CRs are indeed cost-comparable. Another approach is to compare annual costs over a period of time within an organization to determine whether its own costs, evaluated during the postimplementation phase of SLC, have gone beyond those of other budgets within the organization.

When evaluating CR costs, one can sometimes question whether the computer resources are indeed cost-effective. Many times it is difficult to isolate all CR costs when comparing one organization to another. For example, some organizations budget computer paper under individual user area budgets, whereas others allocate it as part of the computer expense.

Response Time

As an organization adds computer applications to existing hardware, there is an increase in computer work time. This increase may have an impact on user VDT response time, i.e., the measured time from when a user enters data in the terminal until the user can enter the next piece of data.

Recent studies have shown that this response time plays a major role in the user's acceptance of computer usage. User frustration is directly correlated with increased response time.

Accommodation of Design Requests

As computers expand within an organization, the need to meet user needs also expands. One approach to systems evaluation and follow-up is to determine the extent to which the applications are capable of meeting new information needs and mandatory changes. Often, prepared reports are part of an application and making changes is so cumbersome, costly, or time-consuming that users develop other ways to meet their needs, specifically using manual methods. A reevaluation of how end-users meet their data needs, as described in Chapter 4, can reveal an application that has not changed to meet the organization's expanded needs.

Systems Use Analysis

The systems evaluation and follow-up can include the amount of time that the user spends using the computer. Evaluation of hardware reports that summarize the amount of time spent using a VDT or printer can lead to a CCRM or UCRM investigating whether an area has too many or not enough VDTs. Possibly, the physical location of the VDTs or printers is a problem. Identifying the fact that an expensive piece of hardware is not being used effectively is part of the follow-up process.

User Problems and Bugs

A follow-up of an installed application can often reveal user problems or program bugs. These problems may have gone unnoticed because the user did not want to mention the problem again or because another solution has been found.

The Survey

One method to identify system evaluation and follow-up needs is a user survey. The design of the survey form is of utmost importance in evaluating the needs. If the form is not designed properly, the answers will not provide a clear picture of the status of an application and of whether the application or system is changing to meet users' needs. Chapter 8 discusses the user satisfaction critical success factors, which are part of the follow-up process.

Other surveys take place through literature searches. One can compare one's own organization with factors discussed in the literature (Bleich et al. 1985, Blask et al. 1985). Costs and benefits described in publications can be compared to those within one's own organization to determine whether similar costs and benefits are appropriate. Further, articles dealing with the management of specialty clinical applications, such as laboratory, radiology, and medical records, will bring to light other approaches to using and expanding one's own computer resources.

Conclusion

Computer systems play such a vital role in modern organizations that they cannot be designed with haphazard methods. Organizations must use documentation and review techniques to organize the development of their computer systems.

A fundamental procedure of systems analysis is the system life cycle (SLC). This is a step-by-step process in which each phase of computer system development and installation is broken down into steps of understandable size. Decisions can be made at each step as to whether to continue, hold, change, or halt the project. This process controls costs and provides management with checkpoints at which progress can be reviewed.

The system life cycle ensures communications between users, CR staff, and vendors. Each phase of the SLC calls for the completion of specific documents. A project request policy is used to ensure proper allocation of limited computer resource funds and staff.

The availability of a computer user group as a unique resource can assist in obtaining information invaluable in systems planning and decision-making. The knowledge of peers can provide insights gained by experience that normally takes years to obtain.

A work committee is essential to interaction and a highly successful computer system. Through the participation and support of all users and by sharing the workload, a system can be designed, implemented, and maintained to satisfy the user's needs.

Various system and programming development tools are available and, in the SLC, provide effective and beneficial systems. These various CASE and 4GL approaches encourage users to participate in the systems design and development process.

As computer systems are installed, the implementation process must be carefully planned to minimize confusion and to maximize acceptance of the system. Various conversion techniques will provide confidence in the system's timeliness, accuracy, and dependability.

When a system is installed to the user's satisfaction, it must be monitored and maintained. Controls on input, output, and database files will assure management that the system's integrity is being maintained.

The predominant theme throughout the chapter has been interaction. A computer system implemented through user and CR staff teamwork will be effective and meet needs and expectations.

There are many other implementation concerns that should be investigated. This chapter has covered areas that should be considered for review and understanding, thus providing the awareness and confidence necessary for successful implementation decision-making. In the SLC, individual guidelines ensure a protected and high-quality computer system.

Questions and Assignments

1. A member of the user staff is quite knowledgeable in computer programming. She wishes to develop and program an application to collect and analyze data specific to her area. The application will run on the user's microcomputer. What concerns might you express as the area's user computer resource manager? What concerns might the central computer resource manager have? How might the programmer address these issues?
2. There have been times when a central computer resource staff quickly programmed a report based on a user's urgent request. It was later learned that the report was not used. What might be done to avoid this expense of money and time? Discuss ways to determine the scope and need of a new report. Might this discussion determine that the report is no longer needed or that the information is already available?
3. Visit an organization that has recently been through a computer conversion. Ask for a copy of the implementation plan. Compare their approach of selection and implementation with the computer resource life cycle presented in this chapter. Discuss the organization's approach in class.
4. Can you succeed without the systems life cycle? Can you be successful and skip parts of the SLC? What parts and why? Describe the SLC to a UCRM and a CCRM? Do they have another name for the SLC? Does an informal (i.e., nonwritten) approach to the SLC exist?

5. Visit an organization and review their disaster plan for computer resources. If it does not exist in written form, what reasons are offered? Ask the user what he or she would do if the entire computer database were lost? How would the user function? Could the user function? How would the user handle a disaster plan if he or she were not limited by time and money constraints? Discuss the value of data.
6. Computer-aided software engineering (CASE) tools and fourth-generation languages (4GL) are becoming routine in user areas. How have CASE and 4GL increased user interaction and dependence on computer systems? Are computer decision-support systems a direct result of 4GL?

Suggested Readings

Amadio, W. 1989. *Systems development: A practical approach.* Santa Cruz, CA: Mitchell Publishing, Inc.

Austin, C.J. 1988. *Information systems for health services administration,* 3rd ed. Melrose, Park, IL: Health Administration Press.

Ball, M.J., K.J. Hannah, U. Jelger, J. Gerdin, and H. Peterson. 1988. *Nursing informatics: where caring and technology meet.* New York: Springer–Verlag.

Blask, D., J. Cleary, and L. Dux. December 1985. A computerized medical information system—sustaining benefits previously achieved. *Healthcare Computing and Communications* 12: 60–64.

Bleich, H.L., R.F. Beckley, G.L. Horowitz, et al. March 21, 1985. Clinical computing in a teaching hospital. *New England Journal of Medicine.* 312(12): 756–764.

Bradejs, J.F., M.A. Kasowski, and G. Pace. October 4, 1975. Information systems. Part IV: protection of health care confidentiality. *Canadian Medical Association Journal.*

Brooks, D.Y., and M.S. Keplinger. 1981. *Computer programs & data bases: perfecting, protecting & licensing proprietary rights after the 1980 copyright amendments.* New York: Law & Business, Inc., Harcourt Brace Jovanovich Publishers.

Bruce, J.A. 1984. *Privacy and confidentiality of healthcare information.* Chicago: Americal Hospital Publishing.

Clarke, R.T., and C.A. Prins, 1986. *Contemporary systems analysis and design.* Belmont, CA: Wadsworth Publishing Company.

Covvey, H.D., N.H. Craven, and N.H. McAlister. 1985. *Concepts and issues in healthcare computing,* Volume 1. St. Louis: C.V. Mosby Company.

DeMarco, T. 1979. Structured English, in *Structured analysis and systems specification.* Englewood Cliffs, NJ: Prentice–Hall, Inc., pp. 179–213.

Minard, B. August 1987. Growth and change through information management. *Hospital & Health Services Administration* 32(3): 307–318.

Minch, D.A., M.F. Meyer, and R. Eller. May 1, 1982. Information system: audit is the first step in planning. *Hospitals* 85–88.

CHAPTER 7

Centralization and Distribution of Computer Resources

Introduction

Definition

Before discussion on whether the management of computer resources (CRs) should be centralized to one CR staff or distributed to the end-users there should be another definition of "computer resources." This definition classifies computer resources into four categories: (1) management resources, (2) systems analysis and development resources, (3) computer operations resources, and (4) database resources.

The first category, management resources, pertains to the people or areas responsible for planning, policy-setting, and prioritizing the acquisition of applications and hardware and their effect on multiarea utilization. The second category, systems and development resources, includes the staff responsible for the definition, design, selection, programming, and implementation of computer resources. Computer operations resources, the third category, includes the staff responsible for the operation of the computers including the facility, hardware, hardware maintenance, and security of the facility and its computer contents. Database resources are the fourth category, and this includes the staff responsible for the definition, collection, and protection of data. The manner in which these four resources are allocated and managed can determine the extent of centralization and distribution of computer resources.

Extreme Centralization

The extreme of centralization would be all four resources controlled by a central CR staff. In extreme centralization, the usage and management of all computer resources are controlled by a central CR manager and a staff of computer specialists. User areas depend on the CR staff for accessibility to the computers, the software, the databases, and the staff resources.

The argument favoring centralization centers on the efficiencies of economics and control that result from consolidating computers, facilities, databases, and CR professionals under the management of one area and one chief information officer (known as the central computer resource manager (CCRM)).

Extreme Distribution

The extreme of computer resource distribution is when each user area has firsthand and sole control over access to all of its CR needs. Today's technology and the computer literacy of user staff make it possible to select and install computer applications with no need for users to seek outside assistance. Applications such as word processing, spreadsheet, and individual user databases can operate on microcomputers and require minimal operator sophistication. Each department's CR needs are met through application parameters and databases that provide a multitude of features with user-friendly instructions. With extreme distribution, each user is free to make application and hardware decisions independent of other users. The application priorities and selection decisions are handled within each user area. There is no need to consult other users, and application software can be purchased as the user sees fit. The computer is physically located and operated in the user area. Distribution seems to optimize each user's utilization of computer resources according to individual user priorities.

A Compromise

Can all of the organization's computer resources (management, systems development, computer operations, and databases) be handled solely by user areas and still meet the information goals of senior management? Can individual users make optimal use of microcomputers, software, personnel, and facility and database resources? Can the CR be centralized under one area and each user's needs be determined by a CCRM, the senior management, or a steering committee? Can user goals and needs be met in a timely and efficient manner when the needs are determined by others?

The three-dimensional matrix of Figure 7-1 attempts to put into perspective the variety of independent decisions that can be made for each user area and for each application relative to the centralization and distribution questions. The decision matrix shows that, rather than looking at user CR needs only in terms of computer resources, it may be easier to break the

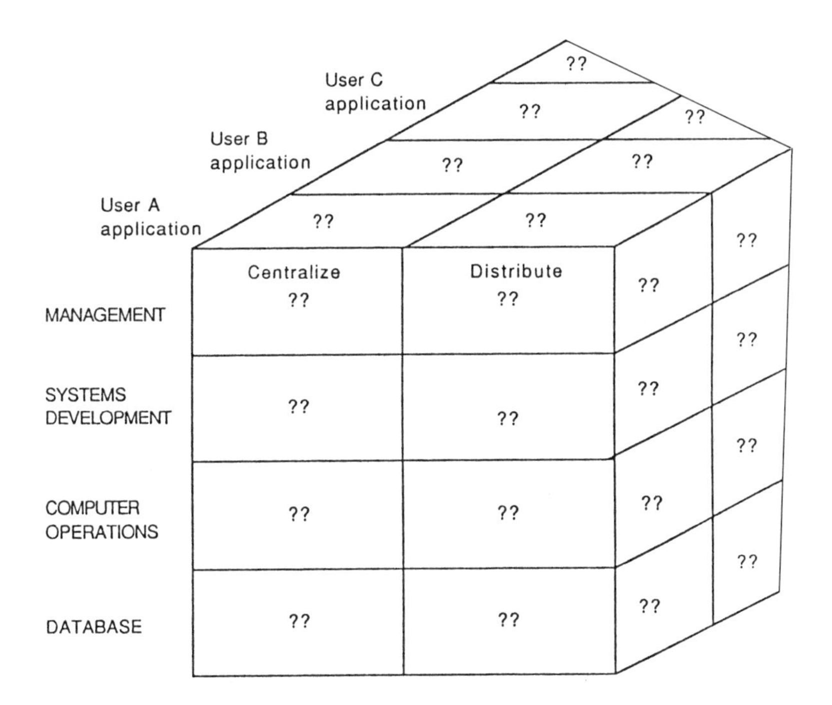

Figure 7-1. A decision matrix to assist in the process of answering the question, "distribute or centralize computer resources?" Reprinted from *Managing Hospital Information Systems* by S. L. Priest, 1982, p. 157, with permission of Aspen Publishers, Inc.

resources into their four components and to set up criteria and make a decision on each resource independent of the other. That is, each user, for each application, can assume responsibility for one, two, three, four, or none of the four categories of CRs.

The Past

Centralization was strongly preferred in the '60s and '70s when computer technology, staff, and budget were essentially limited to financial applications. The few user areas had little or no control over computer resources. In fact, most users did not want this control as they knew little about computers and computers were viewed simply as "data processors" of financial data.

The high cost of computers was not justified for individual users. Computers had to be located in one physical location with a controlled environment. Their technology required special environments with humidity and temperature control and raised floors. In addition, professional CR staff was necessary for programming, systems analysis, and computer operations.

Senior management favored strong central control of all four of the computer resource components. CRs were perceived as being costly and limited in application and as requiring close senior management direction. In fact, senior management knew little about computer applications, only that they were vital to the financial area and were costly in terms of purchase. This meant limiting the growth of the unknown.

The Problem

Centralization can frustrate and isolate users who are prevented from having firsthand control over management and access to computer resources that are vital to their area's productivity and functioning. Users today perceive their requests for new services being ignored or involved in the bureaucracy of a central CR department. They see requests for CR services creating an extensive backlog that is never eliminated because the central CR staff and its limited budget are utilized to maintain existing applications.

Centralization can reduce user flexibility and innovation. Distribution, on the other hand, offers users an opportunity to increase and expand productivity and services. Users' unique needs for decision support systems, office automation, and other productivity systems require individual user management. Centralization, on the other hand, calls for unified planning based on organization-wide information needs.

Alternatives

Today's CR technology offers alternatives to health-care professionals. Computers are used routinely in schools and colleges, and all disciplines of health-care professionals are computer-literate. The mystique of computers has been removed. Microcomputer user-friendly applications provide users the opportunity to define, select, and implement their own applications and systems.

Computer resources can be both distributed and centralized. The low cost of microcomputers and their ease of operation provide the opportunity for nearly every user to manage his or her computer resource destiny. Local area networks (LANs) (electronic linkages that allow multiple computers and applications to communicate) provide the opportunity for these microcomputers to access and use larger computers for shared databases. Microcomputers and LANs can offer the independence and access to data that users and senior management desire.

Microcomputers offer users the ability to manage their own system with no need to interact with other databases and users. LANs provide a method of tying together these microcomputers, word processors, personal computers, electronic mail terminals, portable terminals, electronic filing systems, and central computers. This new technology is the key to today's computer resource management.

Groups of microcomputers offer another alternative to extreme centralization. Physician group practices may have stand-alone systems for patient billing and scheduling, while also communicating daily with a hospital's central computers for ancillary test result retrieval and patient demographic data.

CR Planning

Microcomputers and LANs do not, however, remove the user's responsibility for the effective operation and utilization of CRs and each user's responsibility to meet organization goals and data needs. The potential for excessive and costly duplication of data elements in user areas and the potential for not having vital access to data can require central CR planning.

Senior management, CR managers, and steering and budget committees are confronted with users requesting computer hardware and software that could certainly be implemented and used without the need for direction and assistance from a CR staff. However, decisions to acquire these assets can have a profound effect on an organization's capital and expense budgets and a user's ability to interface information needs with other users. Considerable thought and planning must be given to how each computer resource request should be managed, utilized, and implemented.

These alternatives offer solutions to the question of distribution versus centralization of CRs. The hardware and software technology of today's computer resources challenge senior and user management with an opportunity for innovative planning and utilization.

The Management Resource

The rapid growth and availability of computer technology for user and senior management information needs require review of the question of who should be responsible for the management of computer resources. The past mandate for central planning and management of CRs is now subject to change. CRs no longer need to be solely centralized. The management and utilization of CRs can certainly be assumed by user areas. Management resource concerns include selecting computer hardware and software and ensuring adherence to CR policies. The presence or lack of CR management can hinder a user area's productivity, can cause excessive financial expenditures, can result in underutilized CRs, and can limit the ability to meet both user and senior management decision-making data needs. The degree of CR responsibility that a user can assume relates to management style, organization needs, area productivity, financial status, and experience with CRs.

An Argument for Central Management

The realization that information is a vital ingredient for good management and is a corporate resource that must be managed argues strongly for centralized control over information and the many databases that are available with individual microcomputer applications. The increasing complexity of having to make timely decisions for organizational planning requires central access to user productivity statistics. Decisions about CR budgets and resource allocation must be made. Having the information needed to make these decisions requires a central database fed by compatible systems with common data.

User CR managers must be aware of the need to meet external information requests from outside their area. This external environment includes not only other end-users, but also areas outside the organization such as the government (regulatory reporting). These external data needs are only one aspect of the information needs that complicate today's healthcare environment.

An Argument for Distributed Management

Clearly, today's low-cost microcomputers can place computer power in the hands of every user. Powerful and versatile microcomputers in user areas are operating independent of centralized control and management. Today's technology provides not merely a faster and less costly means of meeting organizational information needs, but also a vehicle for totally new ways in which users and staff can operate.

Apart from cost savings, benefits from the distribution of the management resources include the user's ability to manage information locally. The ultimate benefactor is the receiver of services, as more timely and detailed information can be provided.

A distributive approach to CR management can improve a user's operational efficiency. Computers used solely for individual user applications provide control over resources that directly support the user's area. In addition, a user with its own computer has protection against being affected by organization-wide hardware failures.

The Solution

The solution to meeting the growing demands for distributive CR management can be found by maintaining a centralized CR management resource responsible for developing organization-wide CR policies and network planning. If central CR managers are to assume this role, however, they must be as supportive of the end-user as possible, enabling the user to operate within a comfortable mode. This means giving the end-users as much control and authority over the computer resources as they have over other end-user responsibilities. CR management must organize solely to support the user so that, barring very unusual circumstances, the localized systems and operation resources cannot fail under the user's direction.

We are now faced with the dichotomy of an organization deciding on the one hand that, with limited exceptions, all information technology must be under the control of a centralized CR area. At the other extreme is the move to an organizational structure in which the central CR manager has no line accountability or control over the bulk of the installed computers. The likelihood is that more organizations will find themselves positioned naturally somewhere between the two extremes.

Central CR managers must give up some control over elements of system specification and design, hardware acquisition, data input, and project scheduling. The CCRM will have reduced control over the systems and operations resources, but a much greater involvement in the information needs required for broad areas of organizational decision-making and a clearly defined administrative mandate regarding CR policy and implementation.

Freed from the systems and operation functions, the CCRM can concentrate on the end results for which all of the elaborate technology has been developed: the management and use of information (Warner et al. 1984). Senior management has recognized that, in information, they have a new kind of asset at their command that requires management.

Technological Communication Issues

Future technological changes will most certainly diminish the role of a central CR staff from the perspective of hardware and software utilization. However, from the perspective of networking and service, the central CR staff will still have a major role.

Communications technology for computer interfacing and networking can be controlled and managed by a centralized CR management. Each new generation of computers has increased the importance and responsibilities of this central management resource, which has made decisions concerning the centralization and distribution of CRs more frequent and difficult. Even when extensive data processing operations report to local users, there must be strong central direction and control from a central CR manager. A central CR planning perspective must exist whether an organization uses outside computer vendors and services or has its own central CR staff.

User areas can justify microcomputer costs and need. However, users need a central CR policy to avoid the mistake of acquiring computers that are not compatible with the organization's strategic business plan and the central CR plan.

Experience has demonstrated that tremendous costs are associated with maintaining independent systems that are not used to capacity, store redundant data, and do not network with other computers or databases. Vendors further complicate this distributed management issue as they approach users directly with a turnkey microcomputer, and users purchase services without considering other end-users and organizational needs. Current technology favors central CR planning and control of the logistics of the selection and acquisition of software and hardware resources.

Standards

This centralized approach to CR management can result in strict standards in areas under central control and low or even nonexistent standards in user areas. To avoid this distressing situation, the CR manager must retain sufficient authority to enforce the necessary compliance among users. Standards for data definitions, software applications, file formats, and microcomputer brands must be provided by CR management, and their use must be enforced through budgets and senior management support.

Shared Resources

Users must be educated in the opportunities provided through centralized applications and routines, so they may be effectively shared among all users. This, along with a reasonable amount of systems evaluation and auditing, will help reduce the redundancy of user efforts and the duplication of hardware, software, and staff costs. This evaluation includes the review of computer resource planning and requirements for all end-users. Thus, uniformity and transferability of common systems are maintained.

The Mandate

Directly or indirectly, central CR management must help users achieve the results that they have set out to achieve. The CCRM must have an administrative mandate to guide the spread of computer resources throughout the organization. The CCRM must establish a central planning and management policy for organizational and division-wide system activities so that distributive development work is coordinated. The CCRM must see that systems are designed to respond easily to organization changes as well as to the utilization of new technology advancement. The systems must be designed to respond to specific local needs while maintaining organization-wide hardware and software compatibility.

Central CR management must train users to accept responsibility for the specification and operation of their systems. The management must further demonstrate to users through the interaction techniques of Chapter 3 that data are also an organizational resource to be shared by all. These CR management endeavors will reduce the duplication of user efforts by eliminating the design and support of excessive multiple database systems.

The central CR management must work to develop the skills of user staffs in the usage of systems analysis and operation techniques and must work with them to assign priorities that agree with organization-wide needs and priorities. CR management must control data security and privacy in an organization that will most likely have a combination of centralized and distributive systems and operations resources.

Systems Resources

Responsibility

As organizations become more comfortable with and dependent on microcomputers, users and CR staff can share the responsibility for selecting, installing, and even programming software applications. Interaction between users and the CR staff will always take place, but the determination of who controls the system development resource can depend on user experience and organization needs. Sometimes users will be in sole control of the systems development resource, sometimes control will be in the hands of the central CR staff, and there will be times when control will be shared.

User-friendly fourth-generation languages (4GL) and structured techniques (CASE) allow users to assume many of the systems and programming responsibilities previously performed only by a central CR staff. The result is systems and programming resources that can be both centralized and distributed. However, distribution of the systems and development resource to individual user areas, especially program development, must be carefully planned and coordinated. This responsibility should be assumed only by users proficient at understanding and defining their specific area's needs.

Caution must be exercised when distributing the system and programming resource. Without central CR coordination, distribution can result in a myriad of operating systems, 4GLs, and databases and can lead to organization-wide incompatibilities and restricted user and application interfaces.

There are some users who will write programs to aid them in their unique operations and to provide user-specific information. They will rely on this computer output, and management will rely on their valid programs. But there is no guarantee that their program controls are complete and have been validated. Required controls such as proper documentation and the use of test data are the same, regardless of whether users or the central CR staff are maintaining the microcomputer system.

The responsibility for auditing user-developed programs that are used to provide decision-making information can be shared with a central CR staff, a computer resource support center staff, or an internal auditor. The integrity of data and information from unaudited programs should be verified if these programs are to be used for decision-making functions.

Generally, individual user programming development should be discouraged or at least limited. Most users will use vendor- or central CR staff-developed software. If programming is done within a user area, it must be closely monitored to make sure that the programs are properly documented according to established standards. Experience has shown that users have traditionally done a poor job on documentation. This should be scary for user management. User-developed programs are usually known only by few persons within the user area. It can be disastrous for an area that depends on these programs when the person who has done the program is not available to address program problems and updates. It cannot be overemphasized that user programming efforts should be a last choice and should be approached with caution.

Minicase 1: Nonsupported Software

An example of an attempt to both use vendor-provided software and enhance this software by the user staff, without adhering to program and documentation standards, demonstrates the disasters that can occur if the systems development resource is not managed properly. A user purchased software directly from a vendor without questioning who was to provide updates and changes to the software. After the application was installed, it was learned that the programming updates were supplied by a company 500 miles away and in a language unique to that vendor! The department then decided to modify the vendor's software itself.

The staff maintained no documentation of changes that were made. In fact, the programming staff in the user area consisted of one individual with experience on a home microcomputer. This person then left the organization and, when mandated changes were necessary to the software, it was realized that nobody in the department knew how to make changes or even whether any documentation existed. (It did not!) The vendor's geographic distance made it difficult to get immediate on-site assistance. Furthermore, because the organization had made changes to the vendor's software, the vendor would not guarantee the software. In addition, the vendor's financial position was precarious and the long-term survival of the company was questionable!

This near disaster could have been avoided in several ways. First, the user could have selected a package written in a language known to the central CR staff. This would have protected the department in case the vendor was not available because of distance or being out of business. The department manager could have insisted that documentation be provided by the programmer and reviewed by other people in the department or even the central CR staff. The disaster could also have been avoided if the selected package had been supported locally.

Minicase 2: User Priorities

This example illustrates how distributing responsibility for the systems and programming resource to users could have avoided user frustrations. An organization had centralized its systems and programming staff. User departments could do no systems development on their own. CR priorities were set by the central CR staff and the steering committee and were often in conflict with user priorities. User requests were usually given such a low priority that they were essentially not done. This left department managers frustrated over not receiving services that they deemed to be essential to their department's operation. Why did the CR department exist in the first place if it could not satisfy a user department request? The usage of CRs was restricted. In addition, the users perceived that their departments' productivity was constrained as CR resources could not be considered as a practical alternative to increase productivity.

This example is cited because the demands on many centralized CR staffs have increased to the point where user requests must be answered with alternatives other than "your request has to wait its turn." This problem could have been solved by evaluating the requests to determine whether a microcomputer under the control of an innovative and ambitious department could satisfy the department's requests. A user with a unique need may increase productivity with microcomputers and their applications. Distribution of the systems and development resources on an application by application basis to those users who are capable of handling the resources must be a viable alternative considered for all user requests.

Avoiding the Pitfalls

An organization can avoid many systems development pitfalls when the central CR staff develops microcomputer and software standards for end-users who manage their system development resource. The central staff can be a consultant to users. Using this combined centralized and distributed approach allows many of the systems and programming responsibilities to be handled by users themselves (i.e., the distributive approach), which maintains the independence desired by users. At the same time, the CR staff still maintains control over software standards and documentation (i.e., the centralized approach).

The CR experience of the user area (its track record in managing previous systems development resources) must be considered when deciding to centralize or distribute this resource. A user area that has not maintained documentation and adhered to other development standards should not be allowed to manage the system development resource.

Communication Standards

Centrally developed communication standards and policies can minimize communication problems after hardware and software selection, as when users must share or use information through other microcomputers and communication networks. The task of interfacing a mixed and uncoordinated arrangement of various brands of microcomputers and application and operating software with a local area network can be just too complicated and expensive to attempt. As with any project, the greater the difficulty, the more chance of delays, problems, and errors. In essence, the project of combining nonstandard hardware and software becomes impractical.

Maintaining standards for the microcomputer, peripheral equipment such as printers and terminals, and operating systems increases the potential for future and current interfacing of applications, data, equipment, and staff. Users can then select from microcomputer brands and operating systems that support the organization's CR long-range plan. Standards also allow ease of exchange of staff, hardware components, and software from one computer and user to another for purposes of backup and continued operation.

Documentation Standards

Documentation for systems development is mandated for all areas regardless of whether the resources are centralized or distributed. Documentation standards include user instructions, program logic and flow, and other material necessary for someone other than the user who is intimately familiar with an operation to maintain it. A central CRs staff can monitor adherence to documentation with periodic reviews. Proper documentation assures user areas that their applications will be understood by incoming staff and supported by the central CRs staff if their assistance is needed.

Vendor Standards

A central CR staff resource can develop standard requests for proposal (RFPs) for vendor services and references. For instance, one standard may be that microcomputer and software maintenance be supplied by a firm located within a 50-mile radius. A central CR area can take advantage of bulk purchase discounts, receive central assistance, and have prompt and reliable vendor service. Other vendor requirements in a RFP may include computer uptime, response time, application support and training, and hardware migration capabilities.

Centralization of the planning and standards for system development can also eliminate software and hardware evaluations and expense for the same application and hardware. Comparing various vendor offerings against the needs of the user will decrease the chance of oversight in selecting a vendor or product that does not meet the user's application and support needs. Selection criteria such as response to equipment problems within 2 hours, scope of support including on-site training, and a vendor's offering of other software packages may be of utmost importance in selection. Selection criteria agreed upon by both user and central CRs staff bring the perspective of user and organization into focus. Centralizing and distributing systems development resources can minimize and eliminate undue frustration and even disaster for both user and CR management and staff.

Software Standards

Programming techniques and program standards can provide more usability and exchange on all computers and operating systems. Program transferability between user areas can provide all users with personnel and hardware backup. A programmer in one user area can support another person's program with fewer learning problems because the programs would be written in the same languages and conform to the same set of standards.

Summary

Questions of centralization and distribution of the systems development resource can leave user and senior management frustrated. There are solid arguments for both considerations. Senior management's concerns are planned control of the resources and standards that will provide for increased and complete data for decision-making. Users, on the other hand, want to maintain control of their own destiny. The solution that satisfies both end-users and senior management is a compromise between centralization and distribution. Central systems development policies and standards should be followed for software and hardware. The standards provide for organization-wide hardware and software transferability. User areas will acquire and develop systems that can be enhanced, improved, and supported within the area. The role of the central staff can be that of system and programming consultants. This consultation can provide applications that meet user priorities, needs, and schedules.

A centralized systems and programming staff can set organization-wide hardware and software standards and policies. It can ensure the proper selection of vendors that meet the needs of the user and the organization. The central staff can do programming and systems analysis for those users who do not manage the system development resources. This marriage of the best of centralization and distribution comes with user and CR interaction.

Computer Operation Resources

The Questions

Should a user area have its own microcomputer, supermicrocomputer, or minicomputer, operate it, and be able to communicate with other computers in the organization? Should the user staff have access to update and receive data from central databases? These questions could be rephrased to ask whether the organization should distribute or centralize computer operations resources. As with discussions on the management and systems development resources, the answers to these questions depend on the organization's CR structure and long-range strategic business and CR plans and the capabilities of the user and central CR staff.

Strategy

The strategy of whether to centralize or distribute the location and operation of an organization's computers can be made independent of the strategy for the management and systems development resources, but with a similar evaluation.

A Central Argument. A centralization strategy will be favored for the organization developing a central database, as this function usually demands large scale processors and space and environment requirements necessary for its unique peripherals and operations. However, this does not exclude the possibility of user-located microcomputers for users. Another argument for a centralized strategy may be the need to reduce redundant, expensive, and space-consuming peripherals, such as high-speed printers and computer-output-microfiche equipment.

A Distributive Argument. The argument that host computers are necessary to run a sophisticated application is fast becoming invalid, as today's microcomputers have processing power similar to that of yesterday's mainframe. The availability, ease of operation, and size of most microcomputers require little, if any, physical renovation of the user area. Most space, electrical, and environmental requirements for microcomputers conform to routine office conditions. This certainly favors distribution.

Local Area Networks

User-operated computers that communicate from multiple offices through a local area network can serve to reduce the workload of a host computer burdened with volumes of transactions produced by multiuser areas. With a distributive and workload sharing approach, much of the processing can be handled locally at the user site with selected data elements transmitted to the host.

Users can do extensive verification of data elements at the user level and transmit only "clean" data to the central database. This eliminates extensive processing at the host computer and allows the user to correct polluted data while the data source is readily available. In addition, users can download data from central computers. Thus, data that have been collected elsewhere can be accessible to users who do not have the responsibility of collecting it themselves.

User Ability and Attitude

The decision to centralize or distribute the operations resource of each user area must be based on the user's ability to operate a microcomputer and apply appropriate operational controls, such as those necessary to maintain data files and program backup. In addition, the user's attitude as a risk taker is a factor. The user must be able to recognize that procedural and policy changes may be necessary to implement and utilize the system effectively. Changes bring a certain degree of risk that some users are not willing to recognize.

Ready Access

The need for ready access to the user's data must also be considered in this decision. A further concern may be the host computer's ability to respond in a timely manner because other users will be using the computer's facilities at the same time. Another consideration is the host's capacity to handle the additional volume increases without degradation in response time.

Communication Costs

The cost of the communications equipment and software should also play a role in the determination process. If a user has to access a central database or databases that are located remotely, then the cost of this communication must be factored into any decision to centralize or distribute the operations resource.

Security

Another determining factor may be data security. A laboratory may need to protect its unverified patient result database and be required to handle its own source collection and data definition. This would suggest distributing the hardware resources to protect access to the databases.

Depending on the organizational environment and outlook toward data protection and privacy, there are security advantages to both centralization and distribution. Having all computers located in one centralized area could be considered an advantage because access to the computer facility and files can be restricted and software and hardware accesses can be closely monitored and controlled. In addition, audit trail reports for file updating and inquiry can be centrally monitored with the appropriate staff.

Another organization may consider centrally located computers to be a disadvantage, as the hardware and files could be easily destroyed or easily accessed if located in one area. An advantage of distributing computer data would be the difficulty presented for unauthorized persons trying to penetrate security features located in multiple locations. The separation of computers would make this task more difficult than if all were stored in one central area.

Uptime

Distributive processing may be preferred when the vulnerability of telephone transmissions or the uptime of a central computer can drastically disrupt a user's operations. For example, if an application is unique to the marketing department, such as the ability to locate and access fund raising accounts, the marketing department may decide that a computer located on-site is preferred to a telephone transmission to a remote location or hardwired to a shared computer. The timeliness and availability of access to financial data specific to that user would not be interrupted by telephone or central processor problems. Thus, geographic remoteness may favor the distribution of the computer operations resource. Furthermore, the critical nature of the application and the need for timely response provide a strong argument for distribution.

The concern for hardware uptime and reliability is a vital factor favoring distribution. The failure of a host computer will affect the total organization. The failure of a user computer affects mainly its user, and the remainder of the organization operates normally. With sound, centralized CR standards and policies for hardware and software, a distributed approach using similar brand computers can sometimes provide backup to another user, a luxury not often affordable with high-priced central computers.

Past Experiences

An organization's past computer operations experience with central and user operations resources can affect the decision to centralize or distribute the operations resource to a user area. If the centralized operations resource is considered by management and user areas to be highly responsive to both user and management needs, this factor would favor continued centralization of the resource. Indeed, if this operations staff is user-oriented, it would tend to listen to user requests and respond quickly. However, if the user staff has had previous success with its own computer operations, this might influence the decision toward distribution.

Timeliness

Distributing computer hardware resources to user areas lets the users respond more quickly to needs of scheduling, report generation and report reruns, and changes in VDT screen layouts and formats. The user's computer schedule can be set to satisfy user needs rather than to conform to the availability of host computers.

A conflict between a user's routine schedule and the host's schedule can occur when a host cannot operate because it must transfer data to its own backup files. With some central computers, host computer backup time could mean that essential users will be without computer services during their unique peak hours. Laboratory and pharmacy distribution schedules would have to adjust to the computer backup schedule. If scheduled downtime is required with a user's own computer, the user can adjust the downtime schedule to meet the user's own unique needs.

Costs

The cost of microcomputers is small compared to the cost of large scale minicomputers and mainframe computers. Moreover, distributed computers can be phased into an organization-wide development process and installed only when users are both operationally and financially ready. Host computers that are purchased to satisfy capacity and response needs of five years hence are difficult to cost-justify for the initial years of implementation.

Summary

In summary, the question of whether to centralize or distribute computer operation resources must be looked at from the perspective of senior management goals and user area needs. An argument against complete distribution is that, the more independent systems the organization has, the more chances of a failure through loss of management control. However, distribution allows users to control their own operations.

Each user request for computer hardware must be considered on its individual merits. Hardware and software replacements and additions should not be made simply to meet current state-of-the-art technology, but only after approval is given through cost/benefit analyses.

Database Resources

The Past

Traditionally, system/programming resources included responsibility for the design and definition of all of the organization's databases. These databases were constructed to be part of the application. However, today's database resources can be considered separate from the system development resources.

Control

This separation of resources affects the determination of who controls and updates an application's databases, while preserving data security and integrity. A central database administration can control and monitor the usage and application of multiple databases, reducing the need to store the same data in redundant database files. The same data can then be accessed by many different applications and report generators. End-users can have control over their own databases, and at the same time the organization can have centralized control over a critical corporate asset—data—through a database administration that coordinates and plans the distribution and sharing of the central database resources.

An Organizational Resource

Database technology has progressed so that managing data as a corporate resource (separate from the systems development resource) must be the goal of every organization. Management of data as an organization resource encompasses not only structuring and organizing a multitude of subject databases, but also coordinating and planning source data acquisition to maintain the contents of those databases in a current and accurate state. With this approach, a central data administration function is responsible for ensuring that the necessary source data are made available to maintain those databases that will be accessed by each new application being developed.

Subject Databases

The basic concept of managing data as an organization resource, separate from user applications, has not always been determined in terms of delineation of responsibility between database administrators, systems/programming staff, and users. If data can be organized around subjects, instead of being tailored to individual application uses, the resultant structure can be more easily controlled and shared by everyone. The process of considering databases as separate resources based on data subject involves more consideration than traditional systems design. The separation between management of organization data and user applications that use the information must be clear.

When a project is being planned to service one group of user activities but needs data from a source in another user area, it no longer makes sense for the systems development staff to determine how that source data will be collected and provided. The organization and management of organization data becomes the responsibility of a central database administration. However, application development can still be within the systems development resource, as there is now a difference in the way systems and data structures are developed.

As multiple applications often share the same data, the systems development resource cannot be responsible for capturing the same source data. The central data resource administration is in a position to track and schedule all of the organization's source data collection requirements and to coordinate source data availability with project priorities and scheduling.

User Education

Users involved with database environments should be aware of their role in the organization. James Martin (1981) has published many texts that present simple explanations of the database environment.

Systems Development Resource Responsibilities

The systems development resource will perform the detailed systems data analysis and will define views of the data that must be made available. In this way, the systems development resource is still responsible for identifying the logical views of the data that are required by a particular application, without dictating the design of the organization level subject database. With the framework of subject databases and their data entities, the data administration can then integrate the logical views of data required by an application with those of other applications to create a composite organizational view of data developed over time. Logical views of data can then be translated into physical database definition by data administration.

Data Updates

A key factor in planning for a new application is deciding where and when the source data will be collected. If the system does not collect its own data, some other system will have to acquire it. In a true database environment, there is no longer a need to combine source data collection and usage under the same computer system design.

The 80/20 Rule

A general rule of thumb holds that 80% of information generated within a user area will be used in the local environment, with 20% of the data being shared outside. For example, general accounting has many data requirements unique to the accounting area that require continual updating and accessing by the accounting staff alone. However, the department may also generate data that are pertinent to other departments and that must be made accessible to them via a central database.

In this situation, the organization may utilize microcomputers in the financial office that allow real-time access to a host computer and employee database as well as provide the ability to download data from other subject databases in order to utilize spreadsheet and decision support routines. Selected data elements can also be transferred from the microcomputer to the central database.

Availability and Integrity

Source data availability and integrity may now become a major factor in prioritization of system development projects as the data must be available, or made available, through another resource. This delineation between subject databases and application responsibility is fundamental to the concept of shared subject databases, which is to organize and manage data in such a way that it is available to all who need it.

Security

Database administration may also be distributed to various users. Users with a need to control their own databases and provide unique data security and integrity should be given the opportunity to manage a database entirely separate from the central databases. This could include utilizing various central subject databases to feed the user-managed database with selected elements in addition to source data provided locally. The utilization of microcomputers and local area networks offers this opportunity to control one's own database and to download data from centrally managed subject databases.

The Decision

The decision to centralize or distribute the management of subject databases depends on the availability of that data to other applications, the capability of that area to collect source data and maintain its integrity, and the usage of that data in other areas of the organization. For instance, a public relations department may require its own unique database, independent of other subject databases existing in the organization. The decision may be to allow this user to handle its own database administration. However, if the usage or source of these data also lies within other areas or other areas need access to these data, then maintaining the database through a central administration may be a necessary decision.

Senior Management Involvement

Subject databases and their methodologies are solutions to technical problems. They cannot resolve management problems. They cannot be used to implement solutions to problems caused by users not willing to cooperate and share databases.

Before the development of subject databases, most successful computer resource scenarios have consisted of automating existing business applications that included unique databases such as accounting and payroll. In most cases, however, these automated systems have not really changed anything but a few operating procedures.

The implementation of shared subject databases is going to require basic changes in the way users, CR staff, and senior management view the organization, its operation, and their relationships to both. If senior management, users, and CR staff are able to see the operation of the organization as a whole and recognize that end-user management and information management are inseparable, centralized and shared subject databases will be successful. In organizations in which this is not the case, nothing is really going to change, no matter how good the technology becomes. If senior management does not pave the way and support the concept of shared data resources, then the technology alone will fail. A subject database resource decision to centralize or distribute the responsibility and management of the data resource is dependent on senior management involvement, user sophistication, unique user needs, and overall organization data needs and security.

Computer Resource Support Centers

The Bridge

The need for a computer resource support center (CRSC) evolved because of the introduction of user-friendly technology and the need of central CR management to support this technology in a manner that does not hinder user access to it. Users cannot be deterred from "doing their own thing," whereas the central CR staff still has to maintain corporate data integrity and the utilization of this valuable corporate resource.

A CRSC provides a bridge between CRs and end-users who require automation. The center provides user training and consultation on selected vendor products to aid users in effectively utilizing and retrieving information. The end-users are executives, planners, managers, and office personnel.

The introduction of user-friendly technology such as personal computers, interactive systems, decision support systems, interactive graphics, database report generators, and office automation is making the CRSC a necessary part of the CR structure. However, new user-friendly technology is not the sole reason to establish a CRSC.

The Problem

Traditionally, the major responsibility for providing computer-based information needs, education, and training rested with the central CRs staff as part of its responsibility to install traditional data processing information systems such as payroll. Problems arise when the central CRs staff tries to maintain existing systems and focus on solving old user problems while users are being made aware that long-awaited solutions may be as simple as "doing it ourselves."

The situation is further complicated because 80 to 100% of the central CR systems development resources are generally dedicated to maintaining and enhancing existing systems, and this leaves little time to devote to individual user requests. This has caused user request backlogs that can extend as far back as three or more years. Under these conditions, it is not surprising that both user and CR staff welcomed an alternative.

The Mission

The mission of the CRSC is to allow authorized users at all levels within the organization to use computer technology to satisfy their information requirements. The result is better and more timely information for decision-making, improved CR attention toward organization-wide needs, more timely utilization and retrieval of information, cost reductions and avoidance, and increased office productivity.

The Components

The components of a CRSC include decision support systems that allow users to ask "what if" questions using data centrally located, rapid 4GLs for users to write their own applications, and color graphics. Microcomputers provide users with an opportunity to utilize data at an end-user level instead of being restricted to divisional or corporate-wide data. The CRSC can evaluate new user-friendly technology and software applications.

The Benefits

The CRSC enhances the effectiveness of the CR organization. With the reduction of user requests (as users either write or purchase their own software), the CR staff can spend more time on developing and enhancing new organization-wide applications and reducing existing backlogs.

Staff

A key to a successful CRSC is its staff. The staff should bring a strong user perspective to the CRSC, while relying on the CR staff for its technical assistance. This section's responsibility is to bridge the gap between traditional CRs and office automation and to put the tools for information retrieval directly into the hands of the decision maker.

The CRSC concept must be promoted to the users so that users do not think that the CR staff is simply handing them responsibility that originally was the CR staff's. It is important for the CRSC to be staffed by people who can understand user needs and, through training sessions and site visits (and success stories), make the user aware of the opportunities and assistance that can be provided by decision support systems and other user-friendly applications.

Some organizations include database administration as part of the CRSC responsibility. However, database administration and the CRSC as defined in this chapter are separate areas. To maximize the usefulness of each area, they should be kept distinct.

Office Automation

Discussion of centralizing and distributing information resources would not be complete without including office automation (OA) and the question of its management.

Definition

OA may be defined as the process of integrating computers and communications technology with human patterns of office work. Opportunities for OA include word processing, spreadsheet and graphics, data base, electronic mail, video conferences, calender management, and personal files.

The Question

Should OA be centralized under the CR structure or be the sole responsibility of the end-user? Previously, users could act as autonomous buyers of microcomputers and user-friendly software because OA was associated solely with word processing (WP), but now the leading edge of OA demands a return to centralized planning and decision-making. OA, characterized by advanced communications networks, will call for new, organization-wide standardization and coordination on a level beyond that of the ordinary user staff.

OA History

OA's brief history began with word processing, where it was considered the concern of the end-user. Users and CR staff viewed word processing solely as a secretarial tool and not as part of an automated system that would eventually be just one feature of OA. However, with the growth of OA applications and new computer technology, organizations have realized that OA must be centrally coordinated and administratively controlled.

However, a dilemma has resulted—the OA expertise may lie with the end-user in many organizations. Hence, many organizations may face the question of whether to centralize the OA responsibility under the CR staff (where perhaps there is little, if any, OA knowledge) or to continue to distribute OA responsibility to one or more users.

OA and Word Processing

To many users, OA is synonymous with word processing and in many cases represents their sole foray into the field of electronic data manipulation and storage. This situation could result in various opinions on the extent of CR involvement when a user is selecting OA equipment when its usage will be limited to essentially word processing functions. These discussions depend on whether one looks at OA from the user's present viewpoint alone or as an ingredient of future OA routines that will have organization-wide use.

This discussion takes the stance that the selection and usage of word processing equipment should, at a minimum, be brought to the attention of the CR staff for advice and appropriate assistance in selection. This policy will minimize the duplication of data storage and prepare the user for the opportunities that will become available when OA is integrated with other host systems.

Control

The structure in which OA functions will differ according to the existing organizational framework. One OA structure might be limited to WP and utilize an organizational scheme of a word processing pool under the CR area, where user requests for WP services are sent. Another could be a distributed approach where a host computer or computers are located in the CR area, but visual display terminals (VDTs) and printers are given to each user area for its own use.

Standardization

Regardless of whether user needs are restricted strictly to WP and regardless of the extensiveness of OA, organizations should restrict brands of desktop computers, VDTs, and printers from which the user can choose. Operating system standards should be established so that, if multiuser communication is in future plans (as with local area networks), integration problems will be minimized.

Having the CR staff review OA equipment can mean significant user savings and cost avoidance. The CR staff will be aware of OA equipment compatible with in-house hardware and can avoid acquiring unnecessary and noncompatible hardware and software. Furthermore, vendors who provide current software needs may have OA software that can often be acquired at significant savings and run on existing hardware. For instance, a current in-house minicomputer or host computer may be able to handle

WP software and require only a minimal cost increase for additional VDTs and printers. This alternative may be more satisfactory than stand-alone WP equipment, even without the involvement of other OA applications.

It is possible that existing central CR capabilities can offer many options to the user staff not available with stand-alone equipment. For instance, there can be access to existing CR data files and the potential for organization-wide electronic mail communication.

It will be wise for the user to ensure that any stand-alone system has the ability to communicate with the organization's host computers, as users will surely need to communicate with the organization's other computers. In addition, many of the concerns and parameters discussed in Chapters 4 and 5 for selection of hardware and software, such as file backup and restart capabilities, apply when choosing OA equipment.

OA Standards

A concern when integrating OA and CR applications is that, at present, there are no standards and structure in OA to ensure that all OA software is compatible with multiple vendor standards. The disciplines of data processing will have to be inserted into the world of OA before a successful integration can be accomplished and many of the ideas discussed here achieved. The refinement of local area network technology is an approach that will integrate varied hardware and software brands.

OA and Computer Resources

The options made available by sharing data files between OA and computer resource applications can be very beneficial to both the user and the CR areas. For instance, in a hospital setting the medical record department can use word processing in preparing the patient-physician case summary. The physician can review the transcription using the VDT; a light pen can enable the physician to sign the dictation and then secure its text with a key password. The existing file can then be transferred to optical disks along with the laboratory results and other ancillary reports, thus eliminating paper needs and drastically reducing the size of the medical record. These options are available with the sharing of host processors by both OA and CR applications or when multiple processors can effectively communicate.

Research applications could involve the storage of tabular data on a host processor and the retrieval of that information for manipulation and graphic presentation on a microcomputer located elsewhere. An OA/payroll application file could contain names and addresses useful for generating letters by the organization and being delivered electronically anywhere in the organization. Further, the confidentiality of this mail can be protected with secret passwords and area identification clearances.

OA is playing an increasing role in the utilization of host and user databases. For instance, a secretary can inquire into executive calendar files and schedule a meeting for multiple users without having to make repeat telephone calls trying to identify a common available date. With an electronic meeting scheduler, the secretary can establish a preferred date and have the system inquire as to the availability of attendees. If it is determined that the preferred people can attend, the system will automatically schedule the appropriate date in each attendee's file. The system may even ask the attendees to confirm their expected attendance.

Stand-Alone OA

The acquisition of a stand-alone OA system can be a very complex process. In this regard, the question of managerial responsibility for the equipment acquisition is of secondary importance. The vendor negotiation process is complex and rife with pitfalls for the novice.

There are usually a number of hidden costs that can substantially increase the base expenditure. Aside from the initial outlay for the basic equipment, a maintenance contract is a major cost item that must be considered.

The cost of additional storage space (whether soft disk or otherwise) must be carefully assessed for its long-term financial impact. Add-on features such as noise hoods and continuous form feeders for printers constitute considerable additional costs.

Many OA computer systems have optional software capabilities such as statistical or engineering packages that should be reviewed for their cost savings or loss potential. Installation fees, extra cable needs, static mats, disk filing systems, office furniture to accommodate the units, and labor costs for necessary renovations in multiple VDT environments are among the many concerns that experienced CR staffs have faced.

CR Assistance

The user need not proceed by trial and error. In essence, users are acquiring very specialized computers, and there is no reason to ignore the expertise of people in their institution who have been in this situation before. Any CR staff that has waded through the morass of vendor proposals, contracts, claims, and promises that is part of any major acquisition can give invaluable advice to the user in this stage of the process.

Purchase or Lease

It is also advantageous for the user to keep in mind that outright purchase of OA equipment is only one of the options. In an atmosphere where the development of technology far outstrips its practical application, it might be far wiser for a user area to lease rather than buy OA equipment. The "state-of-the-art system" purchased for many thousands of dollars today might be sadly outmoded in a short period. CR involvement here is not dependent on the actual administrative control of the OA system; it is just a matter of common sense. The institution has consultants at its disposal who can guide the uninitiated through the contract process.

Shared Drawbacks

There are drawbacks to the integration of CR and OA systems. Shared central processing unit time means shared "downtime" as well, and the user can be left without a system when hardware and software technical problems arise even if they are not system-related.

Vendor Specialization

As in other technologies, specialization in OA leads to expertise. A vendor dealing in OA only will offer the user a wider range of options that are immediately available. It is likely that the procedures for using the equipment will be more refined and oriented to the operator who is not familiar with CR concepts. Training of the operator and support of the unit will be more customized. Maintenance of equipment is always a concern, and an OA vendor should be able to provide it quickly and efficiently.

Final Analysis

In the final analysis, the users must determine their real needs. If users are interested in accessing other databases and want to utilize the full potential of office automation, they should carefully consider OA/CR integration. On the other hand, it is important to avoid excessive "blue sky" planning if the need for shared databases and communication does not exist.

This section has provided some answers to the question of the centralization or distribution of OA because each organization must evaluate its own OA needs and in-house expertise. Whatever decision is reached, however, the CR staff can surely make the user aware of available options and the potential integration of OA and CR applications.

Conclusion

Independent Decisions

The decision to centralize or distribute computer resources can be made independently for the management, systems development, database, and computer operations functions. Furthermore, a decision can be made independently for each user area and each application need. Each resource decision must be considered in light of its ability to serve both organization and user CR needs. User area characteristics will influence the centralization/distribution decision and the CR capabilities of each user's management.

Unique Applications

Users with unique application needs generally favor a decision to distribute information resources. Whereas those users with applications that relate to other users usually support a decision to centralize.

Control

Distributed CRs represent an exciting management option, but "distributed" cannot be synonymous with "random". Senior management must always be in control of each resource, regardless of whether it is distributed or centralized.

Management Interest

Frequently, a critical factor in the decision relates to the level of interest that senior management shows in CRs. The attitudes of steering committees, the CCRM, and user management can affect the responsiveness of CRs to user requests and cost-benefit priorities. A senior management with little interest in CRs may tend to favor CR decisions being made at user area or division levels. If not controlled properly, these decisions could later result in frustration when data are recognized as an organization's resource, but cannot be utilized because of no planned standardization for interdivision hardware and software development.

A senior management that recognizes the potential of the data resource will carefully consider the long-range plans of both the organization and the CR area. Decisions of whether to centralize or distribute resources will relate to a user's need for CR responsiveness and the user's internal ability to manage, staff, and budget to meet the need.

Planning

Each organization must plan carefully how computer resources will be used in the future. Along with general plans, the CR management must promulgate policies establishing how computer resources will support user area computer systems and needs. Only with such plans and policies can the organization assure itself that a user area computer system is capable of integration into an organization-wide network.

Standards

Reasonable standardization of microcomputer hardware and software can benefit the distributed and centralized staffs in systems development, databases, and computer operations resources. The centralized management function can then play a higher role in data management and become an integral part of the organization-wide planning and decision-making process.

Computer Resource Support Center

The introduction of CRSC to assist users in meeting their information needs can play an essential role in allowing departments to focus more on traditional CR applications. A CRSC can allow users quicker and more detailed control over their information usage.

Office Automation

User areas considering office automation (OA) should consult with the CR staff on the many exciting opportunities offered by the integration of OA and traditional data processing applications. The points made in this chapter can be strongly associated with many of the views presented in other chapters. Long-range planning and project selection play an important role in decisions to centralize or distribute the computer resource responsibility.

Questions and Assignments

1. As data become an asset to an organization, its management becomes essential. How should senior management organize the staff to ensure proper use and review of data? How does a database administrator (DBA) play a role in this function? Do

most organizations today have a DBA? Why not? Who is the best person to assume this role? Why?

2. A head nurse has been offered a microcomputer for the preparation of her monthly statistics. The present method requires manual preparation of the statistics and is quite time-consuming. A physician on the staff has offered to donate a used brand Z microcomputer. Brand Z is not supported by the computer resource department, but there are other departments that have used brand Z. A new microcomputer, one that is supported by the CR staff, costs about $4,400. The preparation of nursing statistics is the only application to be used on the microcomputer.

   You are the nurse's supervisor. Should she accept the gift? Explain your answer.

   You are the central computer resource manager. Should she accept the gift? Explain.

   Are there other alternatives that will provide the needed statistics?

Suggested Readings

Austin, C.J. 1988. *Information systems for health services administration.* Ann Arbor, MI: Health Administration Press.

Buchanan, J.R., and R.G. Linowes. July–August 1980. Understanding distributed data processing. *Harvard Business Review* 58: 143–153.

Buchanan, J.R., and R.G. Linowes. September–October 1980. Making distributed data processing work. *Harvard Business Review* 58: 143–161.

Kroenke, D.M., and K.M. Dolan. 1988. *Database processing: fundamentals, design and implementation.* Chicago: SRA.

Martin, J. 1981. *An end user's guide to data base.* Englewood Cliffs, NJ: Prentice–Hall, Inc.

Warner, D.M., J.C. Holloway, and K.L. Grazier. 1984. *Decision making and control for health administration: the management of quantitative analysis.* Ann Arbor, MI: Health Administration Press.

CHAPTER 8

Ongoing Computer Resource Management

Introduction

Success Can Lead to Further Challenges

The development of successful computer resources (CRs) is a never-ending process. Once a satisfied user proclaims the benefits of computerization, other areas begin to demand similar recognition and services. As more areas acknowledge that CR services can further increase their effectiveness and productivity, they will request CRs for assistance. In essence, success so diligently achieved can mean an increase in demand for CR services; if not managed properly, this demand can lead to costly and ineffective use of CRs.

A problem can occur when satisfied users recognize additional uses for CR services, while at the same time new users are requesting CR services, and all areas seem to have an immediate need. A central computer resource manager can become frustrated attempting to satisfy this demand for increased CR services and stay within the capabilities of the CR staff, equipment, and budget, while trying to maintain the philosophy of being a service-oriented function.

Squandered Resources

Another situation causing CR concern is when end-user expense and staff budgets seem to be increasing at unacceptable rates, apparently beyond their control. The previous allocation of computer resources to these areas had been justified through both user estimates and feasibility studies that predicted significant savings in expense and staff hours. Where are the savings that had been expected? Were CRs squandered by a user that did not quantify, document, and thus effectively utilize any of the resulting savings?

A Formal Planning Process

Such dilemmas may be faced by users and CR managers (i.e., the central computer resource managers and user computer resource managers) and their staffs if each does not develop a formal planning process that addresses the utilization of CRs. This need for comprehensive CR planning has been mentioned throughout the text. Any CR plan must align its goals with those of the organization's long-range strategic business plan.

Effective CR planning can minimize expensive crash programs and avoid a crisis orientation. It can tie together and integrate the many subsystems and tasks required of users and the CR staff. It establishes and projects the funds, facilities, and expertise required for future development. It is a significant factor in meeting short- and long-range goals and can act as a motivating force for the people using the CR because it indicates where they are going. Both short- and long-range planning are emphasized in this chapter because they are clearly important elements in the continuation of a successful CR.

Priorities

Another element that affects the spirit in which CRs are perceived by end-users is the method by which CR needs are prioritized within the organization. Project priority is obviously an important part of short- and long-range planning. To many users, the priority assigned to their project is an indication of how their responsibility is perceived within the organization. The method by which projects are selected and how this method is understood by the user are important to the continual success of CRs. Prioritizing can also affect the cooperation of the user staff with central CR staff on current and future projects.

Postimplementation Studies

The third element necessary to justify CRs is postimplementation studies, which measure items such as cost savings, cost avoidance, improved quality of patient care, and other tangible and intangible benefits. These benefits can be measured only after the CRs have been allocated and utilized. Essentially, postimplementation studies show whether the benefits obtained exceeded the cost of using the resources.

Critical Success Factors

As the various CRs become integrated into the organization's daily routine, the CR managers are still responsible for the successes and failures of the CRs. The information necessary to monitor the functioning of computer resources is available in varying degrees of detail in most user areas. The difference between CR managers who have become leaders in both their organization and industry and managers who continually struggle with day-to-day operations is that the leaders have learned to identify CR critical success factors (CSFs) (Bullen and Rockart 1981, Rockart and Bullen 1986) and have concentrated on managing them.

The CR manager must identify selected key indicators to assist in performance evaluation and decision-making. Each manager must identify CRs that are not cost-effective and performing to expectations. Potential problems must be recognized before they become critical. Two key CSF areas are cost and user satisfaction. The four elements of successful CRs—planning, prioritizing, performing postimplementation studies, and identifying critical success factors—are discussed in the following sections.

The Long-Range CR Plan

The Organization Plan

First there must be an organization-wide long-range strategic business plan. One must know where the organization wants to be in two to five years before any CR long-range plan can be developed. Without an organization plan, CR development and utilization has no direction.

Purpose

A long-range CR plan provides general strategies that focus on usage and development of the CR for a two- to five-year period. Essentially, the CR plan is a reaction to the organization's overall goals and long-range strategic business plans and, as the organization's objectives and needs change, so do the priorities established in the CR plan.

The CR plan has three primary purposes. First, it should give senior management control over the growth of the computer resources. As discussed in Chapter 7, the centralization and distribution of resources must occur in an orderly manner to prevent situations in which senior management has little or no control over the growth and use of CRs throughout the organization. Second, the plan will allow the user areas to anticipate the acquisition of the CR. The rising cost of staff, hardware, software, and facility renovation must be prepared for and funds must be allocated to ensure the planned acquisition. Third, the long-range CR plan affects end-user short-range goals and objectives and provides guidelines for end-users to work with each other.

Content of the Plan

A typical CR plan will discuss application implementation schedules and priorities, funding, state-of-the-art technology, staffing, physical needs, and management CR policies. Plans may address expected cost/benefit measurements and other indicators that will be used to monitor the progress and success of the plan, such as CR budget and staffing levels. Figure 8-1 shows the questions that must be addressed during the development of the CR long-range plan.

Preparation for the Plan

There are many processes that have to occur before the actual written plan is prepared. The user areas must determine their CR needs and decide whether these needs are aligned with those of the organization. This can be accomplished through review of the organization's long-range strategic business plan and through users being involved and updated in current organization happenings. CR users can participate in various committees and be put on circulation lists for planning memos.

Industry Concerns

CR staff must be up-to-date with state-of-the-art CR applications and techniques. CR staff should review user journals. Membership in CR-oriented organizations will provide both the central CR and the user staffs with an awareness of current topics of importance, such as federal and state legislation, vendor offerings, and other CR planning sources. Meetings of vocation-oriented organizations, such as the Healthcare Financial Management Association (HFMA) and the College of American Pathologists (CAP) can be attended by CR managers to anticipate and recognize present and future concerns and problems that will be addressed through computer resources.

Figure 8-1. CR long-range planning questions.

1. Is the Plan aligned with organization-wide goals and strategic business plans?
2. Does the Plan relate to the scope of and relationships among other CR applications?
3. Should the Plan address cost and funding concerns?
4. Should facility needs (user and CR area) be considered for hardware and staff location?
5. Should staffing changes be considered?
6. What expertise (user and CR staff) is required for carrying out the Plan?
7. Should the Plan consider short-range plans of other departments?
8. Has the user had sufficient input into the Plan, and does the user understand the Plan? (The user does not necessarily have to agree with it!)
9. Are the priorities of applications clear?
10. Are the schedules and milestones realistic?
11. Should risks and backup plans be explained?
12. Are the goals in the Plan obtainable and practical?
13. Is state-of-the-art technology considered?
14. Are the benefits to be received clear?
15. Are measurements of performance indicated?
16. How frequently should the plan be updated?
17. What methods will be used to educate users before and during the implementation?
18. Should legislative mandates be considered?
19. How will training (user and CR staff) be accomplished?
20. What acquisition method will be used?
21. Are the values and philosophy of management reflected in the Plan?
22. Are any assumptions explained?
23. Should the Plan address CR policies?
24. Does this Plan consider last year's experiences?

Participation in the Organization's CR Strategy

The CR mangers must routinely meet with senior management and provide input in determining the goals and strategies of the organization's strategic business plan in order to have a full perspective on the direction and tone of the CR plan. This involvement will also update senior management on the present state of the art and on the direction of CR development.

Assisting Other Users

CR managers can assist each other in the internal planning process by sharing information and literature on current hardware and software systems particular to their respective interests. This can also be accomplished through formal and informal discussions.

Education

As discussed in Chapter 3, the central CR staff can offer seminars on computer resource concepts and responsibility. This will provide continual exchange of information between users, senior management, and the central CR staff. Such seminars will help to educate the parties to each other's concerns, and will provide insights into potential system problems, as well as other background information necessary before a long-range CR plan can be prepared.

The First Plan

One "how to" protocol for preparing a long-range CR plan is the needs definition approach as discussed in Chapter 4. When preparing the first long-range CR plan and later when revising it, each user's information needs should be surveyed and recognized—regardless of whether these needs will be met by manual or computer methods or by in-house or outside vendors. This approach assures that the entire organization's information needs have been examined and reviewed. Prioritization of these needs can then be done by a steering committee, and these priorities will serve as the foundation of the plan.

An Off-Campus Planning Session

Long-range CR plans should be prepared by both the central CR staff and the user staffs. The plans should be reviewed, updated, and approved at least annually. The revised plans must be routinely shared with all areas.

One approach to finalizing a long-range CR plan is to discuss the items at a steering committee planning session. One can schedule a full one- or two-day session, preferably outside the organization's campus. An off-campus atmosphere and environment will minimize interruptions and allow everyone's complete attention to be focused on the task at hand. These planning sessions should take place annually.

The formal session agenda can begin with evaluating what was done during the past year in achieving the plan's objectives. An end-user was supposed to accomplish certain items by certain dates and with financial returns. Were they achieved, and what changes are necessary to this year's plan so that next time the objectives will be met? In essence, this review of the past is a learning and educational process for the committee. In addition, the review can determine whether the accomplishments were usable and beneficial to the users, senior management, medical staff, community, and patient.

Last year's plan can be evaluated to determine whether it makes sense in the current year. As the plan was prepared last year, revision may be necessary to conform to the organization's and user's current goals, which may be different from last year's. The revisions necessary to bring the plan up-to-date with these current needs and perspectives should be discussed. It is also necessary to bring year two of the plan into the detail stage. The remaining years should also be reviewed and revised if necessary, and a new fifth year should be added.

The agenda for this formal off-site planning session should be carefully prepared before the meeting. All necessary documentation and statistics should be made available to the committee prior to the meeting.

Input to the Plan

When preparing the plan, the CR staff must consider input from all areas in the organization, regardless of each area's current CR needs. All too often, plans are prepared using only input from current end-users. This can result in rebuttal against the plan by nonuser areas that have been thinking about using computer resources, but have been awaiting technological or application advances. These areas should also have input into the plan. Some areas may have concerns about interfacing and using systems developed primarily for other areas. For example, a nurse order system, planned for each nurse unit to order ancillary tests, may be of concern to the dietary department because dietary staff need to be involved in the definition and selection of any system that determines patient preparation orders.

Administrative Policies

Administrative policies that may be included in the plan are the general guidelines for the implementation and selection of organization-wide applications and microcomputers. For example, a plan may specify that all microcomputer purchases be first reviewed and evaluated by the central CR staff. It could further state that stand-alone microcomputers must meet certain networking criteria and have the potential to communicate with other in-house computers.

Environmental Concerns

The long-range plan must recognize existing and future organization environmental plans that will be an influence on the type and scope of computer resources. For example, a nursing home about to merge with another facility may delay expanding its own computer resources until it has time to evaluate the CR staff and resources of the new facility.

General Management Strategy

The effect of personal values of general management and directors regarding planning and strategy must be considered. If medical directors or trustees have more influence on long-range planning than the senior managers, this influence should be reflected in the plan.

Intangible Benefits

The opportunity for intangible long-term benefits can be addressed in the plan. For instance, an office automation system whereby managers can have long-distance conferences televideo may offer minimal cost savings, but for a growing organization the system may aid a turnover problem among senior staff who had been required to perform extensive travel.

Measurements of Performance

The plan should specify objectives and measures of performance that will guide the prioritization and scheduling of future CR applications and strategy. For instance, an organization may quantify reductions in accounts receivable as one criterion for a new application. This criterion may be used to implement an on-line accounts-receivable system with the receivable days being measured in a follow-up study to determine the success of the implemented system.

Time Span of the Plan

It usually is difficult for most organizations to plan more than two to five years into the future given today's financial and legislative climate. In addition, computer hardware and software technology is advancing faster that one's imagination can anticipate. For this reason, many plans address only three years into the future. However, three years sometimes pass quickly. Thus, a typical plan can be developed and divided into three stages. The first stage is relatively detail-oriented and covers at least the next year. This stage may even be the short-range plan. The second stage could have plans that encompass general strategy for the next one to four years, and the third stage a four- to five-year "wish list" that deals in "if we could have anything" topics. Of course, the third stage is extremely "blue sky," but is always the "carrot" that could be considered.

The Final Plan

Approval of the CR plan can come from senior management, the steering committee, the board of directors, and other committees involved with planning of services. The plan acknowledges an agreement on the direction for the organization and for individual user areas. As one goes through the investigative and approval process, there will be revisions and updates as additional input is received and the health-care environment changes. In fact, an approved plan is simply that—a plan. It is subject to change and will serve as a planning outline for other services.

The final CR plan is used by each user area to plan staffing, training, new procedures, and equipment and facilities. The plan should even be used by an area not included in the CR plan so that it will not spend time evaluating systems not included in the organization's future CR plans and funding.

The plan allows end-users to anticipate future directions and services so that they can orient and train their staff. However, one must consider that things do change and the organization will not be a slave to the plan. Even so, the plan will give guidance to the preparation for future developments such that current procedures can be integrated into systems proposed hence. For example, if the central CR department's long-range plan calls for the implementation of a centralized database in three years, the department can consider in the design of current applications the ability to communicate via a local area network in the future.

In addition, a user request for computer resources can be compared to priorities established in the plan. This may result in a request for CR services being delayed because of future plans for a compatible system that may conflict with the request. For example, a request to make an immediate major change to a batch payroll system may be postponed as the CR plan calls for an on-line payroll system in one year. The expenditure of CR resources required to make the current request may not be justified when considered in relationship to future plans.

Topics Not in the Plan

Not all requests will be included in the approved plan. For example, a department may request word processing (WP) services. If the organization has determined that the integration of word processing services is not an organization-wide priority, then the decision to acquire WP may remain within the user department's own long-range plan, even though it is not in the organization's long-range plan.

Summary

The benefits of long-range computer resource planning are that it:

- Integrates CR priorities with the organization's strategic business plan and
- Allows the user and central CR areas to plan for:
  —Timing
  —Facilities
  —Staffing
  —Procedures
  —Budgeting.

The particulars and methods of CR long-range planning certainly will vary from facility to facility, and the listed topics are only guidelines. Figure 8-2 summarizes the various topics that can be addressed. What is most important is that long-range CR plans do exist for the organization and each end-user. Without long-range planning, the benefits of CRs are difficult to achieve and recognize, and the support and funding will not be available.

Short-Range CR Plans

Purpose

There are a variety of approaches to developing short-range CR plans, and these plans can have many names and formats. Generally, these written plans address specific tasks in detail that are to be accomplished within

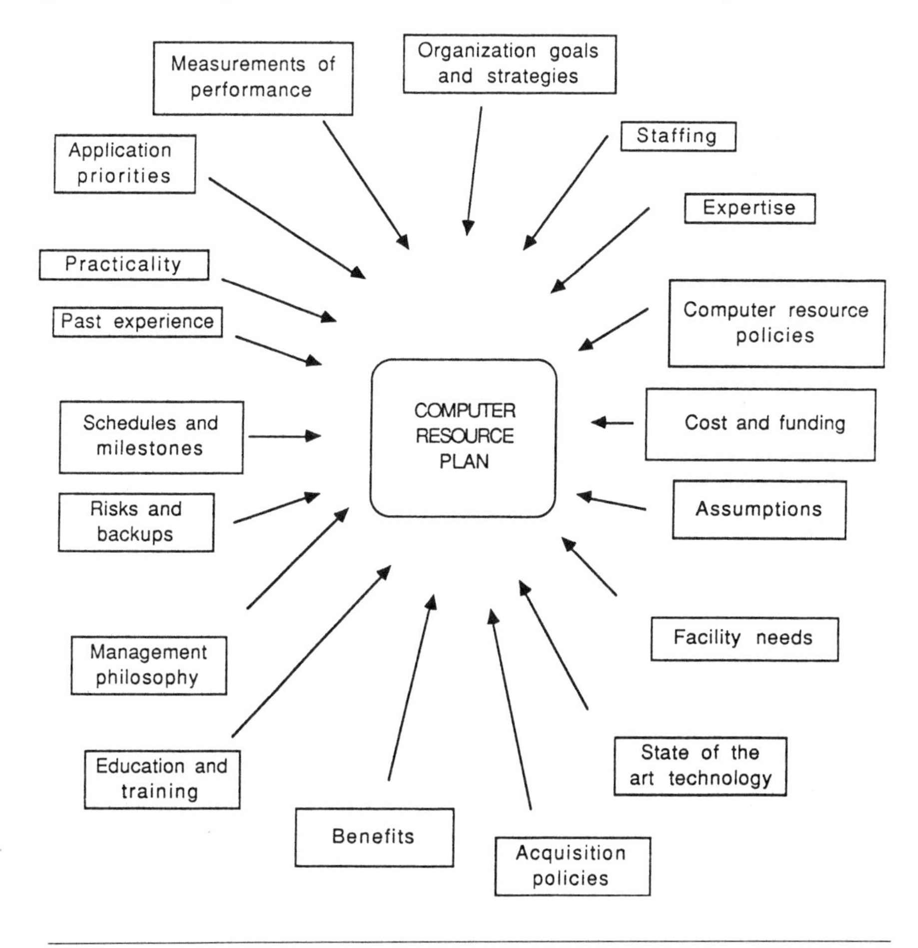

Figure 8-2. The long range computer resource plan.

weekly, monthly, and annual schedules. An effective user of CRs has some type of short-range plan that enables the user to function objectively and to maintain a perspective on its priorities within the organization. Whatever the title of the plan, its purpose is to provide the CCRM and UCRMs with a tool for planning and controlling the direction and application of computer resources and activities.

A Multitude of Plans

End-users usually have a variety of short-range CR plans. For example, a department can maintain a current project schedule. This short-range plan would include a description of current projects and their status in terms of percentage completed and expected completion dates. Further, this plan could include the number of staff-hours and the costs utilized thus far for each project.

A Goal-oriented Plan

A short-range plan may address the CR goals that the user area is expected to reach during the calendar year. This plan would be prepared in conjunction with the current project schedule. It would contain milestones showing the expected cost/benefit measurements for a project: "the completion of project #A is expected to reduce time in the turn around of laboratory test results by 8 hours." The plan can also be used by the CR manager to evaluate the area's annual performance and its ability to estimate expected completion dates and costs.

These plans are generally prepared by the UCRM and are used to monitor the area's monthly and annual accomplishments and progress. Some managers highlight these short-range goals and plans through a bulletin board that displays the annual project plan and current project schedules. A scheduling board can be used to display Gantt charts with expected completion dates for each project, as well as other visual graphic techniques that allow easy review of a project's status and a staff's CR accomplishments.

Summary

An end-user's short-range CR plan must conform to the goals and directions established in the long-range CR plan. The steering committee and the UCRM can use the short-range plan to review the user's progress to date and as an overview of the user's current project status and adherence to the organization and CR long-range plans.

Project Priorities

Who Determines Priorities?

Which CR project request should be scheduled first, if at all? Which project should be delayed until a more appropriate time? Which request should be turned down? Determining project priorities can be cumbersome and frustrating to the CR manager as well as to a steering committee. In addition, the requestor can become frustrated with the attention, or lack of it, being given to his or her project. Textbook theory sometimes simplistically proposes establishing a method that determines priorities based on quantifiable cost/benefit measurements. Further, some may be emphatic that project priorities should always be set by the steering committee, with the CCRM and UCRMs being responsible only for carrying out the priorities of the committee. In reality, there are a variety of methods used to set project priorities.

Steering Committee Priorities and Daily Priorities

Of course, many project priorities are set by the steering committee. This committee is comprised of general management and user representatives and provides the direction for computer resources to serve the interests of the organization as a whole. However, there are day-to-day decisions that must be made to maintain continuity of CR responsibility.

Using only the steering committee to establish project priorities would drastically hinder the operation of the user area in its objective to provide timely and effective systems to users. Many minor requests would never be submitted by users if approval of the committee was required. An experienced CR manager can gauge the necessity of many of these minor requests without going through formal approval and prioritization procedures. For example, if a department makes a request for a special report and the CCRM knows that it can be accomplished through a database directory change, it is impractical to go through formal review channels. Instead, the project is accomplished within the time demands of the current workload.

Project Workloads

To be responsive to user requests and the setting of project priorities, the CR manager must understand project request and completion rates. Ninety percent of all requests take less than 20 days to implement, 9% take two to 12 staff-months, and 1% take more than 12 months (Sneider 1987). To address this breakdown of project request workload and its effect on the changing daily needs of the organization, one can establish a work request control and priority system that categorizes requests as minor, intermediate, and major projects.

Project Priority Categories

The setting of priorities can usually be classified into three categories: (1) If it's broken, fix it! Thus, if a system has a bug and it is preventing utilization of the system, this system is given top priority. (2) Legislative mandates—if the government mandates tax changes by a certain date, this may necessitate advancement of the priority to meet deadlines. For example, the hospital industry with the introduction of diagnosis-related groups (DRGs) in 1984 was forced to rearrange its CR priorities to meet a legislative mandate. Each organization had to anticipate the financial impact and had no data available to judge the DRG impact. (Now, as DRGs are introduced for outpatients, all health-care facilities will need to have data available to plan their decision-making and strategies—thus, they will need to prioritize new CRs to provide the tools to collect, store, and analyze appropriate outpatient data. (3) The third classification can differ from organization to organization and is arbitrary. Justification can be on the basis of cost, staff, patient quality of care, community relations, etc.

One must set project priorities after considering the CR long-range and short-range plans and available CRs. Priorities can be based on cost savings only. If a project saves in tangible costs more than the cost to implement and maintain it, then the project is given priority.

Priorities Based on a Hot Button

Priorities based on an organization's latest "hot button" may be in response to a corporate mandate to do whatever is necessary to get a share of the market. This would be the CR priority guideline for this year, even though cost savings may be important. In a year of high nursing shortages, marketing nursing opportunities may be the corporate hot button. The focus is on attracting the staff necessary to maintain and expand the organization's services. For other organizations, a freeze on hiring may be the hot button and projects that can produce a reduction in hours or increased utilization of existing staff may be given top priority.

Categorizing Project Priorities

For the category method summarized in Figure 8-3, a minor project may be defined as one taking less than a week of staff effort. An intermediate

Figure 8-3. Categorization of CR project requests versus level of priority decision.

	Priority Decision Made by:		
Request Category	**User CR manager**	**Senior management**	**Steering committee**
Minor (less than one week)	X		
Intermediate (less than four weeks)	X	X	
Major (greater than four weeks)		X	X

project is one that requires less than four staff-weeks of effort, and a major project is a task that requires more than four staff-weeks. With this type of project effort breakdown, the minor and intermediate projects can be prioritized by the CR manager who, with input from the staff, can then schedule the requested project for implementation. If the CR manager does not consider the project to be worth the CR effort, but the requestor does not agree with the manager's evaluation, the project can be further reviewed by senior management. All major projects are prioritized by the steering committee and senior management.

The deadline for a project can automatically determine its priority. For example, if a federally mandated requirement is necessary for payroll on July 1, the priority given to this requirement must reflect this time schedule.

Priority Methods

Whatever system is used to prioritize and select CR projects, it must be designed so that it encourages user requests through timely and fair consideration of the request and allows the CR manager and senior management to monitor the breakdown of the various types of project requests. Thus, the system must make the CR managers, senior management, and steering committee aware of the focus and extent of CR allocation.

Informal Priorities

Priorities can be set according to the prestige of the individual making the request. For example, if the chief executive officer needs a report, then this project may be given a rush priority even if it does not go through the regular priority process. This method should be used infrequently.

Priorities Based on Promotion of CR Services

Formal criteria should be used for prioritizing projects, and most likely these criteria are set by the CR managers and the steering committee. However, there may be other less formal criteria. For instance, an organization just establishing computer resources or one trying to maintain a progressive reputation may decide that, to promote the full usage of CR services, all reasonable requests will be implemented if possible. This will help the CR managers to establish rapport with users and demonstrate an effective available service. As time goes on, this philosophy will need to be changed as the CR managers become deluged with requests.

Availability of Staff Resources

The availability of CR staff resources plays an important role in the setting of project priorities. Is there enough staff available to handle the request within the necessary time frame? Do the people available have the capability of handling the request? For instance, a request to develop an organization's client forecast simulation model may be judged to be too time-consuming or too esoteric for the staff's breadth of knowledge. This project could be given a high priority and the necessary software could be acquired through the services of an outside vendor or the central CR staff.

Cost Priorities

One obvious priority criterion is the cost of allocating CRs for the project versus the expected return in benefits. A request that takes two staff-weeks to complete and saves a half-hour per year of user time may be judged to be impractical. Feasibility studies may also reveal that it is more practical to improve an existing manual system than to utilize limited CRs.

Project Request Procedure

CR project requests can often be initiated through a formal system such as the type of project request form shown in Figure 6-1 of Chapter 6. A form of this type helps to establish in writing the requestor's commitment to the project. Hallway conversations with the CR manager and user do not necessarily mean user commitment. A project that is initiated because of a hallway request can turn into a major project because of lack of user commitment or understanding of the scope of the request. Sometimes, when quickly requested systems or programs are installed, it is learned that the hallway conversation was merely a question and not really a request. This can result in frustration for the CR manager and many wasted staff-hours and resources.

Postimplementation Studies

The Questions

Just as important as long-range plans, short-range plans, and project priorities is the need to identify benefits received from the utilization of CRs (Kralovec and Schatek 1988). A cost/benefit study, also referred to as a return-on-investment study, should take place after every project has been completed. These studies should be carried out after the user has become accustomed to the new procedures and changes. The study can address many questions. Were the economic benefits of the project (e.g., a reduction in radiology staff hours) fully realized? If so, where are these savings now? What are the intangible benefits received from the project? For example, was there an improvement in patient test result delivery time by getting physician orders from the office to the hospital faster? What were the actual costs of CRs compared to the expected costs, and did the actual tangible benefits exceed these costs? Further, can we share the experiences gained from this project with senior management, CR staff, and other users? For example, a method developed to teach users the capabilities of a new on-line system may later be used by other departments. Postimplementation studies add another step to the implementation process, but their importance cannot be overemphasized.

The Justification

Computer resources represent 2 to 5% of an organization's operating expenses (Packer 1987). This investment must be continually justified, but many CR managers find it difficult to allocate time for this task. It is as if the cost of the justification is not worth it. Somehow postaudit evaluations are forgotten or ignored in the clamor to create new and more powerful systems. To ignore postimplementation studies can have serious long-term consequences for the organization.

When organization policy requires that all implemented CR projects have cost/benefit studies and the studies are reported to senior management, the policy can provide a system of checks and balances that hold down superfluous requests for CR projects. A user has to justify expected benefits versus "good to have" applications. To satisfy the ego of a user manager will not be the only reason for implementation. In summary, postimplementation reporting:

- Utilizes bottom line savings,
- Documents savings,
- Confirms the value of CR expense, and
- Provides confidence in CRs for present and future uses.

Minicase 1: Expected versus Received Benefits

A purchasing department's budget was increasing at an unacceptable rate. A microcomputer was purchased and justified by the department on the basis of expected savings in negotiations and an accompanying reduction in budget, but the department was still over budget. A cost/benefit study was not conducted after the system was installed. If it had been, it would have shown that extensive buyer and utilization reports were indeed present, but that the purchasing and user staff had not made efficient use of them. Thus, the expected reports were present, and a postimplementation study would have revealed the staff was not trained in how to use the microcomputer's reporting features effectively.

Parkinson's Law

Parkinson's law states that "work expands to fill the time available for it." This occurs when actual staff-hour savings are absorbed into a user's routine activities without recognition. A project that is expected to save staff-hours can often lose its purpose if not monitored. Users should be required to examine the effectiveness of the CR applications and to isolate benefits and costs.

Baseline Measurements

For a postimplementation cost/benefit analysis to be made, it is necessary to develop baseline measurements before a system is changed or implemented. Measurements should be made in each area used to justify the system. Usually, these initial baseline measurements are identified during the feasibility study.

Minicase 2: Real-time Clinical Benefits Received

One justification for an on-line laboratory clinical system and census system was an expected elimination of misdirected laboratory patient test results for admitted emergency department patients. In the feasibility study, the laboratory, nursing, and emergency departments worked together to document an average of 40 patient laboratory results per day returned directly to the emergency department after the patient had been transferred to an inpatient nursing unit. Further, the rerouting of these test results averaged two hours per day of emergency department staff time and required an average of four telephone calls from nursing units looking for the results. After the new systems had been operating for six months, a second study on misdirected results was made and the results were compared with the first baseline study. The results showed that essentially there were zero misdirected laboratory test results for inpatients admitted via the emergency department. Thus, the cost/benefit follow-up analysis documented the benefits of the new systems in staff-hour savings and in improved patient care due to quicker result reporting.

Minicase 3: Documented Benefits

Demonstrating savings through postimplementation cost/benefit analysis is shown by the case in which undelivered patient meals are returned to the dietary department each day because of patient discharge, transfer, and fasting. Nursing's unusual occurrence reports could further document cases of fasting patients mistakenly given meals, resulting in contaminated or delayed tests. The preimplementation feasibility study may have determined that the reason for these dietary problems was delays in getting accurate patient census, schedules, and dietary information from nursing stations to the dietary department. Thus, this preimplementation study may have justified a new census and dietary application because of expected meal cost savings and improved patient care. After the system has been working for a period of time, a follow-up cost/benefit study could determine the effect of the new system on the dietary problem. The study could show cost savings in terms of meals saved and the long-term effects on average patient stay.

Richard M. Sneider (1987) discusses actual case studies of projected versus actual savings in equipment, labor, and purchases through the use of real-time organization-wide computer resources. The effect on quality of patient care and the economic impact on an organization are documented. Examples of savings in pharmacy, admitting, nursing, and other areas are given. Covvey et al. (1985) give examples of decreasing staff, increasing staff efficiency, reducing turnover, and saving supply costs. Benefits such as fewer telephone calls in nursing and ancillary areas and reallocation of job assignments have been studied. Without such studies, it would be very difficult to take advantage of the changes in staffing schedules and responsibilities.

In another scenario demonstrating the impact of postimplementation studies, a senior manager claimed a savings of 4,160 staff-hours a year through effective usage of computer resources. This savings translated into two staff positions. When this claim was made, however, the administrator responsible for the area required the manager to identify the two employees who were eliminated. In essence, the manager had to show that the staff-hours saved were being allocated to tasks that had not been done previously.

Chapter 11 describes typical items that can be identified through feasibility and justification studies and later reexamined in the cost/benefit postimplementation study. The scenario quantifies savings in nursing, laboratory, pharmacy, patient registration, medical records, dietary, finance, medical staff, and even physician offices. Table 8-1 shows some items that can be measured when quantifying actual cost and staff-hour savings.

Sharing of Studies

Cost/benefit studies should be shared with all users and senior management. All concerned areas will be informed of the effect of the CR, and pride will be instilled in users by showing them and others the fruits of their efforts with a successful and beneficial CR.

Publications

Another method that can be used to report cost/benefit studies is the publication of CR articles in professional journals. This method further promotes pride in CRs, assuring continued upkeep of the system, and serves as continual justification for further usage of CRs.

Serendipitous Benefits

The postimplementation analysis will often reveal benefits not seen in the feasibility study, as well as the absence of benefits that were expected but not realized. For example, an analysis of a recently installed laboratory CR may reveal a significant reduction in telephone calls from the radiology staff because they can now directly access hematology results. Investigation may also reveal unexpected deficiencies in training and implementation methods. Once these deficiencies are recognized, additional CR benefits can often be achieved.

Table 8-1. Typical Quantitative Cost, Staff-Hour, and Unit Measurements.[a]

	Pre	Post	Difference
Average patient registration time (minutes)			
Inpatient			
Private outpatient			
Clinic outpatient			
Emergency area			
Repeat outpatient			
Same day surgery			
Data entry full-time equivalents			
Monthly revenues and volume by user area (Recovery of lost charges)			
Accounts receivable days			
Average number of daily telephone calls to nursing and ancillary areas (looking for patient location and test information)			
Trips per week to deliver requisitions (By user area)			
Full time equivalents by user area			
Reports distributed			
Forms cost by type form			
Wasted meals			
Transfers			
Discharges			
Changes			
Medical record retrievals for discharged patients (to put results into record)			
Minutes spent per user area for pricing			
Pharmacy inventory in $			
Dietary inventory in $			

[a]Numerous variables do affect an institution during a given period, and these variables should be factored out of the "Post" measurements. Examples are marketing ventures, new ancillary services, and patient volume changes.

Reprinted from *Managing Hospital Information Systems* by S. L. Priest, 1982, pp. 192–193, with permission of Aspen Publications, Inc.

Users that do cost/benefit studies continually learn from the experiences gained through the follow-up analysis. This knowledge educates the CR and user staffs for future studies and can even generate new feasibility studies for additional projects.

Summary

Through cost/benefit studies, the presence of CRs is justified.

Critical Success Factors

Satisfaction Success Factors

CR managers must respond to their users in a timely and effective manner. The degree that users are satisfied with CR can be monitored with user satisfaction pulse points.

A CR manager should operate in the same fashion as a company that takes market surveys to test the level of satisfaction with its product. A good product can bring additional sales and recognition for the company. A responsive company that seeks to improve its product enhances company esteem and solidifies its hold on the market. This holds true for successful CR managers.

Low Priority of Satisfaction CSFs. A literature search offers limited information on user satisfaction pulse points. This indicates that CR managers are hesitant to question users on their degree of CR satisfaction.

In an informal survey taken by the author, over 100 CR managers were interviewed for their user satisfaction pulse points. Only five managers had developed routine procedures that monitored user CR satisfaction. The conclusion drawn was that users are generally not asked to evaluate their CR services. Many of the managers' responses were, "if they are not satisfied, they will call me!" This assumes that if there are no complaints the user is satisfied. This assumption may be correct, but it is the author's opinion that complaints are not the sole indicator of dissatisfied users. CR managers seem hesitant to seek user opinions for fear of rocking the boat and discovering problems that they consider to be picayune.

Complaints may not be made by a user who has continually been frustrated with CR services and has turned elsewhere for assistance. However, the CR manager may eventually hear of these complaints when senior management voices concerns over excessive and unanticipated use of outside CR services.

Figure 8-4. User satisfaction questionnaire. Reprinted from *Managing Hospital Information Systems* by S. L. Priest, 1982, p. 146, with permission of Aspen Publishers, Inc.

TO: Computer Resource User

FROM: User Computer Resource Manager

Please indicate the degree of your satisfaction with the computer resources that you are using. Any additional comments that you would care to make would be appreciated.

	Outstanding	Satisfactory	Not Satisfactory	Not Applicable
Time required for new systems development				
Your participation in establishing CR priorities				
Processing of requests to existing systems				
Timeliness of routine reports				
Accuracy of reports				
Response of central CR staff to corrections				
Degree of training				
Your understanding of existing systems				
Formats of existing reports and screens				
System manuals				
Uptime of hardware				
Flexibility of systems				

Comments:

CSF Questionnaires. User satisfaction pulse points can be developed through questionnaires similar to that in Figure 8-4. A CR manager can periodically survey the user staff and develop indicators from the responses. The questions can concern timeliness, accuracy, effectiveness, and cooperation from the central CR staff a well as from themselves. Each question can be assigned a given value, and a total point score can be developed. A minimal point level would warrant further investigation. This technique lets users know that the CCRM and UCRMs are interested and provides a forum so that the CR manager can identify problems early.

CSF Memos. CR managers not wanting a technique as formal as a questionnaire and survey can use something as simple as a memo asking for user comments. Again, the objective is the same, to let users know that the CR manager welcomes their input and concerns and wants to enhance CR services.

CSF Log Books. Another pulse point can be the analysis of an ongoing log book of user complaints and problems. This can be kept by category such as unscheduled access to the CR, machine breakdowns, software bugs, and enhancements. This log will identify outstanding CR issues and their current status.

Level of Services. The CR manager must put user satisfaction pulse points in perspective. If a CR manager attempts to assess user satisfaction without relying on an objective outline, the result can be misleading. For example, a physician could call the CR manager to complain of late laboratory reports. The complaint may be stated so that it seems that all reports from the user area are late. The physician may not realize that, with the exception of this one report, all other reports are on time. If the CR manager provides the end-users with information on the level of CR services received, CR services are put in perspective.

User Sensitivity. In summary, CR managers must be sensitive to their responsibility within the organization and the degree to which CRs provide acceptable services. This sensitivity can be enhanced by developing quantitative user satisfaction pulse points and by informing users of the degree of CR services received.

Cost Success Factors

How much should be spent for CRs? What are reasonable CR costs? CR managers look for rules of thumb and other standards in setting CR budgets, monitoring expenditures for CRs, and determining whether CR costs are high, low, or reasonable.

Unfortunately, there is no one best rule. In reality, judgments on reasonable CR expenditures usually depend on comparisons with organizations and other users offering similar services, as well as an organization's satisfaction with its current level of CR services.

Industry Standards and Reasonable Costs. Organizations today spend 1 to 3% of their operating dollars on computer resources (Packer 1987, Dorenfest 1987). The percentage of end-users within the organization dependent on CRs to meet their productivity and reporting responsibilities has risen significantly, particularly within the hospital industry as a result of diagnosis-related groupings (DRGs). As DRGs or similar cost-containment, monitoring, and utilization systems become required for all health-care industries, providers will be required to make significant investments in computer resources. If history repeats itself, these organizations will cautiously look to each other to determine reasonable computer resource expenditures.

A word of caution when using comparative unit cost methods for CR expenditures. Not all organizations and users budget CR expenses using the same allocation method as to which accounts will be classified as computer resource budgets. For example, the cost for preprinted computer forms used by a billing office may appear in the budget of their department because that department purchases the paper. Other organizations may have the central CR area budget for this item. Thus, in evaluating reasonable costs by looking at similar organizations, one must determine whether all computer costs are being recognized and accounted for under specific computer budgets and are being reported as CR expenditures.

For an organization considering using or expanding computer resources, whether on-site or outside services, the cost comparison figure of the CR expenditures as a percentage of total operating expenditures can be used to provide estimates of the expected cost to provide computer resources. For example, Table 8-2 is an industry cost survey that community hospitals of various bed sizes would use to compare and evaluate computer expenditures. A 220-bed hospital can multiply its total operating expenditures by 2.1% to compare its CR costs to industry averages. In addition, 1 standard deviation can be used to determine a reasonable range of expenditures.

Some organizations prefer to adjust the patient-day cost calculation to reflect ambulatory services by using an additional patient-day for every 3 ambulatory visits or by increasing the patient-days by the percentage of receivables represented by ambulatory services. For instance, if a hospital

Table 8-2. Community hospital operating expenditures for computers by bed size.[a]

Bed Size	% of Total Operating Expenditures		
	1984	1985	1986
Under 100	1.79%	1.49%	1.40%
100–199	1.52%	1.92%	1.94%
200–299	1.99%	2.10%	2.10%
300–399	1.91%	2.17%	2.34%
400–499	1.96%	2.41%	2.38%
500 & above	2.19%	2.36%	2.53%

[a]Reprinted from *The State of the Art in Hospital Information Systems* by Sheldon I. Dorenfest, with permission of Dorenfest & Associates, Ltd., Northbrook, IL.

has 100,000 inpatient-days and 25% of the receivables result from ambulatory patients, then the patient-day figure used in the CR cost per patient-day calculation is 125,000. If this hospital has 100,000 ambulatory visits per year, it could also choose to consider 3 visits equal to 1 patient-day and use a patient-day figure of 133,333. Thus, when one compares CR cost per patient-day with that of other organizations, one must know the calculation method: inpatient-days only, days adjusted by visits, or days adjusted by percentage of ambulatory business.

An organization may be concerned that it has not made enough of an investment in a particular resource, such as the central CR support staff. More detailed industry averages that present CR expenditures by staff percentages could help determine how much similar organizations invest in their support staff. Statistics are also available for such details as hardware, software, and supplies (Dorenfest 1987, Packer 1987). An organization concerned that it is spending too heavily in one area can also make valuable use of industry statistics.

The selection of an indicator for CR expenditures depends on the availability of comparison statistics and the organization's use of the statistic.

The Budget. Budgets and cost control procedures for CRs are essential if organizations are to maintain, improve, and justify their levels of productivity. All cost decisions, actions, and results are ultimately reflected in a CR budget. The budgeting process produces numerous pulse points for utilizing cost and revenue for both the organization and user areas. A CR budget can be set up to monitor costs associated with the central CR and user staffs, and some costs can be broken down by function or product within each area.

Typically, the budget reflects expected and actual expenses on a continuous basis, allowing managers to identify pulse points that compare the costs and performance against forecasted expenses and actual savings. The budget allows realistic, equitable, and identifiable distribution of CR costs reflected by services rendered or costs incurred. The comparison of actual to forecasted costs is one way to determine expectations of upcoming budgets and future costs.

Project Costs. Budgets can be assigned to unique computer resource applications. For example, one can establish a budget for the medical records department to switch from microfiching patient records to the utilization of optical disk technology, and actual expenditures can be measured against the budget. Job performance and the costs and staff hours expended in preparing for the new technology can be accountable by the individual responsible for managing and implementing the new technology.

Personnel Costs. Personnel costs can be compared to industry averages. For example, 26% of CR expenditures is attributed to personnel. If your organization is spending 50%, there may be reason to review the services being provided that make your organization different from the industry average. The efficient utilization of user staffs may also be reflected in a cost pulse point, such as measuring the ratio of dollars saved per staff cost.

Hardware and Software Costs. One pulse point is dollars spent for hardware compared to the situation in similar industries. Another is software costs, both one-time and ongoing, and the cost of software maintenance by the vendor. A pulse point may be software expenditures over the last few years versus what was actually received in benefits from this investment.

Communication Costs. The latest cost element in computer resources is teleprocessing costs. The use of satellites, telephones, and other networking methods to communicate both within and outside an organization is sharply rising as information is made available without concern for the boundaries of oceans and outer space. Pulse points can be identified to monitor communication costs versus the benefits derived, such as reduced travel expenses and faster decisions from geographically separated staff who can meet via teleconference and facsimile.

Graphic Presentations. Examining expenditure pulse points alone may not allow ready determination of whether expenditures are above or below budgets and expectations. The numbers themselves may not be enough to define trends, which is essential for effective pulse points. A technique that works well and is widely used because of its simplicity is to graph the pulse points. Figure 8-5 illustrates such a graph where a pulse point is viewed over time. In the bar graph example illustrated, the facility's computer resource expenditures as a percentage of total operating expenditures is compared to a national average for a similar size facility. Each year the manager enters the previous year's actual CR expenditures and plots the actual expenditures against an industry average. The graph in this example shows that the facility's computer resource expenditures are well within the industry average. Presenting this display to the steering committee and senior management would give a clear picture of actual costs compared to industry averages. Line, bar, pie, and stack graphs are easily prepared using microcomputer spreadsheet and graphic software and downloading data from a central database financial system.

Charging for CR Services. One of the most controversial issues in computer resource management and cost accounting is the question of charging for CR services. Should the central CR services be provided free to each end-user? Should those who use CR services pay for them? Is cost charge-back an effective pulse point or a headache for all concerned? Will it inhibit the usage of CR services?

A charge-back system should be implemented only after thought has been given to how it will affect the organization. Management must first clearly define what it hopes to achieve. If charge-backs are used, they must be both for cost accounting and as a tool for managing the utilization of CRs.

A charge system can report the costs of central CR services to the user and maintain an account of central staff hours spent on a development. Often, a user does not realize the hours and costs devoted to system development and changes. Whether charge-backs are used or not, reporting these figures to user managers brings into focus the financial and time costs associated with computer resources.

Application Development Costs. A look at the CR budget of Facility XYZ may show very little being spent for new systems development. The level of spending for new systems and development may be barely adequate to maintain the current level of system support. As a result, this facility cannot emphasize systems development; however, their long-range strategic plan calls for new CRs.

This dichotomy may be eliminated with an increase in the CR budget for new developments. A budget increase may allow the facility to increase its ability to develop new systems by 100 to 200%! This increase in development costs can be monitored using pulse points to identify quanti-

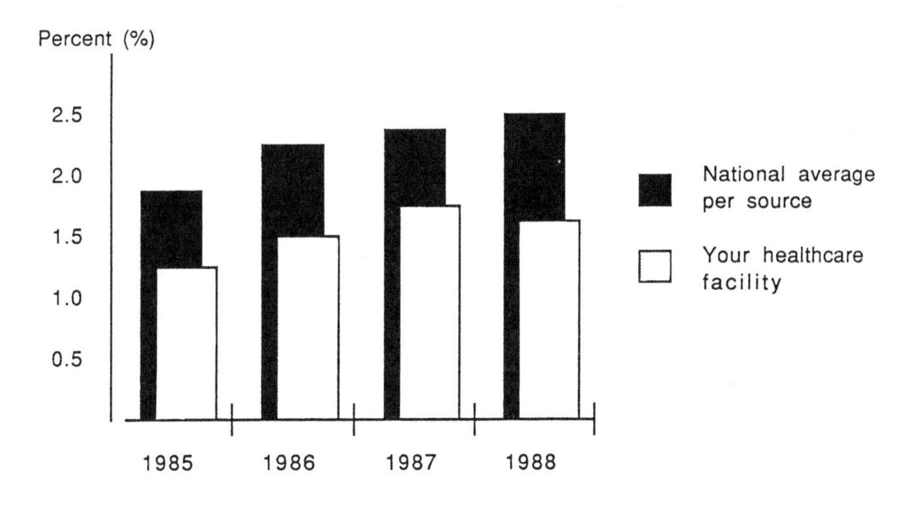

Figure 8-5. Graphic presentation of computer resource expenditures as a percentage of total operating expenditures.

tative benefits and savings in user productivity. As organizations develop plans for real-time patient care and clinical data reporting systems and expect these new CRs to have an impact on services and end-user productivity, they will need to provide adequate funding to ensure planned systems development.

Cost versus Effectiveness. When industry indicators are used to determine reasonable expenditures, the result of these expenditures must be put into perspective. For example, two industry indicators of hospital CR expenditures are the CR expenditure per patient-day and the CR cost per patient-bed. However, these comparative units do not reflect the ambulatory services portion of the hospital's business, and most certainly these figures do not indicate the impact on users, patients, and medical staff.

If a facility has limited ambulatory services and payroll is its only CR application, the CR expenditures may be $1.00 per patient-day. A second facility with complete ambulatory services and numerous CR applications, including payroll, may have a cost per patient-day of $2.00. Which facility is better utilizing its CRs? Without knowing each facility's ambulatory service load and the productivity and patient care effectiveness of their CRs, one cannot answer this question. This example relates costs within hospitals. However, published industry cost indicators for all health-care organizations are available through various sources. For effective use of cost indicators, CR budgets must reflect an ability to offer comparative calculation methods. These published indicators must be used only as guidelines. Expected benefits in decision-making, data, staff productivity, and quality services must be the determinants of CR expenditures.

Weighted Values for End-User Effectiveness. Cost CSF indicators do not provide a measure of the effectiveness of the end-user computer application. For instance, patient-day cost alone will not differentiate the extensiveness, productivity, and cost-effectiveness of an automated laboratory system. This can only be determined with a comparative unit that relates costs to application effectiveness. This comparative unit can then be used by a facility to determine the effectiveness of CR services and thus to substantiate or change the use of computer resources and its CR budget.

Weighted unit value systems recognize that application ABC may contribute more to an organization than application XYZ. However, weighted systems are not widely used today, as it is difficult to have universal agreement on weights, their specifications, and essential applications. This agreement can only result when a national organization becomes committed to collecting data and publishing national statistics. A value system may be developed as federal and state regulations attempt to delineate information resource costs.

Organizations, however, can develop their own weighting system and send surveys to other institutions for comparison. A comparative unit calculation can be developed based on numerical weights for each application, resulting in a unit value cost per weight. The method can be further explained by example. An organization with a payroll application could receive a maximal weight value of five for a payroll system that meets certain specifications. A preventive maintenance system might have a maximal weight of three (because the organization may classify it as a nice, but not essential application), but be given a value of two because it met only part of the specifications. Dividing the CR expenditures by the sum of all the user's application weights will provide a cost per weight. The organization could then compare this figure with figures for similar size organizations and, hopefully, soon-to-be-published industry-weighted statistics.

Cost-Effectiveness. Cost indicators can be used to plan, justify, and evaluate CR expenditures. When reviewing CR expenditures, however, the main concern should be the effectiveness and utilization of services provided through CRs. Literature that explains the experiences of others in evaluating the effect of CR expenditures on economic, personnel, and user areas can play a vital role in determining the direction, extent, and effectiveness of one's CRs (Sneider 1987, Austin 1988).

An increase in CR expenditures may be justified by a comparable decrease in staff and costs in a user area. Likewise, a CR expenditure made only to be comparable with another organization or to be state-of-the-art should always be questioned. Each CR manager must identify one or two cost pulse points that reflect the priority CR expenditures.

Conclusion

The Organizational Plan

Long-range and short-range CR plans must not be developed in a vacuum. First, the organization must have its own long-range strategic business plan. The CR plans can then be developed in concert with and supportive of the organization plan.

Continual Success

The continual success of CR requires long-range and short-range planning, project selection and priorities, cost/benefit studies, and utilization of critical success factors. The proper use of these management tools can provide efficient utilization and allocation of CR resources. The CR manager must promote these tools through user education and interaction.

Planning

Long-range and short-range CR plans are necessary before CR managers can properly allocate CR resources to assist the organization and end-users with their present and future needs. Plans allow managers to interact with potential users and assist in attaining their present and future information needs.

Long-Range and Short-Range Plans. An organization must consider that short-term plans may have long-term impacts that can be diametrically opposed to the organization's strategic business plan and goals. An organization must recognize that new CR applications and technologies will be developed and must begin to decide how it will deal with them. The long-range plan allows such a focus. The organization's CR plans must be developed in conjunction with user areas. The content of these plans should include projects to be undertaken and their prioritization, cost/benefit analysis, scope and relationship of projects, staffing and facility requirements versus available resources, external and internal plan assumptions, overall organization strategies and guidelines, budget projections, schedules and milestones, and risks and backup plans.

Priorities and Planning. Project priorities and selection must also coincide with the organization's short- and long-range CR plans. Projects not within the plans should not be prioritized, as the focus of the CR should be on agreed-upon organization and end-user goals. This section discussed project priority methods based on feasibility studies, peer group pressure, management style, long-range plans, and other criteria. Priorities can be set by steering committees, user computer resource managers, central computer resource managers, or senior management depending on the priority criteria established.

Postimplementation Studies, Plans, and Priorities

Postimplementation studies are an essential step in the computer system life cycle. These studies evaluate the result of proper planning and project selection. They determine whether the plan's expectations were achieved, whether CR services are being used properly, and whether CR allocations were justified.

The CR Image

This chapter has demonstrated a need for CR policies and procedures regarding the usage and justification of CRs. Senior management must be continually aware of the effect of the allocated resources and must require documented justification for CR expenditures. The public relations role of UCRMs and CCRMs can be assisted through cost/benefit studies and the publication of professional journal articles. The importance of CR manager interaction is displayed and documented through the application of long-range planning, project prioritization, and cost/benefit studies.

Critical Success Factors

Cost and user satisfaction pulse points can be used for monitoring and managing the effectiveness of the CR. Although there are many statistics available, the successful manager will select only two or three for regular review. In addition, a pulse point will change as the priorities of the end-user area and organization change.

Pulse points should monitor the degree to which the CR is meeting end-user responsibilities. Pulse points should be developed so that they are easy to review and require a minimum of collection effort.

Satisfaction CSFs. Pulse points for user satisfaction have yet to be recognized as critical by most CR managers. The development of user satisfaction pulse points should be a priority for all CR managers.

Cost CSFs. Cost pulse points are necessary to respond to the many financial and budget constraints placed on the organization and its various components. The innovative CR manager will use cost pulse points to recognize and justify services.

Summary

Many of the examples and the methods discussed in this chapter can be associated with topics in Chapter 7 on the centralization and distribution of CR. Readers interested in other cost/benefit studies and methods are encouraged to read studies in professional and other literature sources. CR and user staff interaction is essential to planning and justifying the allocation and acquisition of CR resources.

Questions and Assignments

1. Critical success factors (CSFs) are essential in all aspects of health-care management. Interview an office manager and ask for a definition of what is critical to the success of the manager's job. What key data elements do managers monitor to determine whether a function is in control or getting out of control? How are these elements collected and on what frequency? Be sure to read this chapter first and have a clear understanding of what a CSF is. Users may not know the CSF term, but they will know it by your definition.
2. Organizations sometimes have a difficult time preparing a long-range computer resource plan. Many do not even have an organization long-range strategic business plan. How does an organization without a long-range strategic business plan go about preparing one? If an organization long-range plan does not exist and the computer resource department is approached about expansion, how does the department respond?

Suggested Readings

Austin, C.J. 1988. *Information systems for health services administration.* Ann Arbor, MI: Health Administration Press.

Bullen, C.V., and J.F. Rockart. 1981. A primer on critical success factors. Cambridge, MA: Center for Information Systems Research, Massachusetts Institute of Technology, Sloan School of Management.

Covvey, H.D., N.H. Craven, and N.H. McAlister. 1985. *Concepts and issues in health care computing*. St. Louis: C.V. Mosby.

Dorenfest, S.I. 1987. *The state of the art in hospital information systems.* Northbrook, IL: Dorenfest and Associates.

Henderson, J.C., J.F. Rockart, and J.G. Sifonis. September 1984. A planning methodology for integrating management support systems. Cambridge, MA: Center for Information Systems Research, Massachusetts Institute of Technology.

Kralovec, J., and L. Schatek. Winter 1988. Cost benefits realization: Stanford University Hospital blends management engineering and information system resources. *Journal of the Healthcare Information and Management Systems Society* 2(1):4–5.

Packer, C.L. August 1984. A comparison of hospital data processing costs. *Hospitals* 58(15):83–86.

Packer, C.L. December 20, 1987. Information management: Data processing budgets jump during 1987. *Hospitals* 61(24):60.

Rockart, J.F., and C.V. Bullen. 1986. *The rise of managerial computing*. Homewood, IL: Dow Jones-Irwin.

Sneider, R.M. 1987. *Management guide to health care information systems.* Rockville, MD: Aspen Publishers.

CHAPTER 9

Diary of an Integrated Computer Resource

Introduction

Chapters 1 through 8 discuss principles and concepts as they relate to defining, selecting, implementing, and managing computer resources. These principles apply to all health-care providers: hospitals, long-term care facilities, home health agencies, nutrition services, mental health agencies, satellite clinics, and physician's offices. The scenario that follows demonstrates many of these principles as we follow Shauntim Hospital through a process of implementing and identifying the benefits of a real-time shared database system. The discussion is from the perspective of various medical disciplines (Priest et al. 1988).

The hospital's trustees have recognized a need to review their current state of automation and to develop a computer resource plan that is in compliance with the hospital's long-range strategic business plans. The scenario begins with Shauntim Hospital evaluating its information needs and whether they can best be met by automation. The hospital will go through the needs and priority process and identify vendors who can meet its needs and goals. The hospital's medical staff also have access to the central database from their offices.

The Shauntim Hospital has installed a real-time shared database computer system. With a shared database, departments use common data entered at many sources. The system integrates various software applications, referred to as modules, and combines them into a single system so that a person with an authorized password sitting at a visual display terminal (VDT) can look at complete patient data as a single entity even though the data may have been provided by various departments using individualized software.

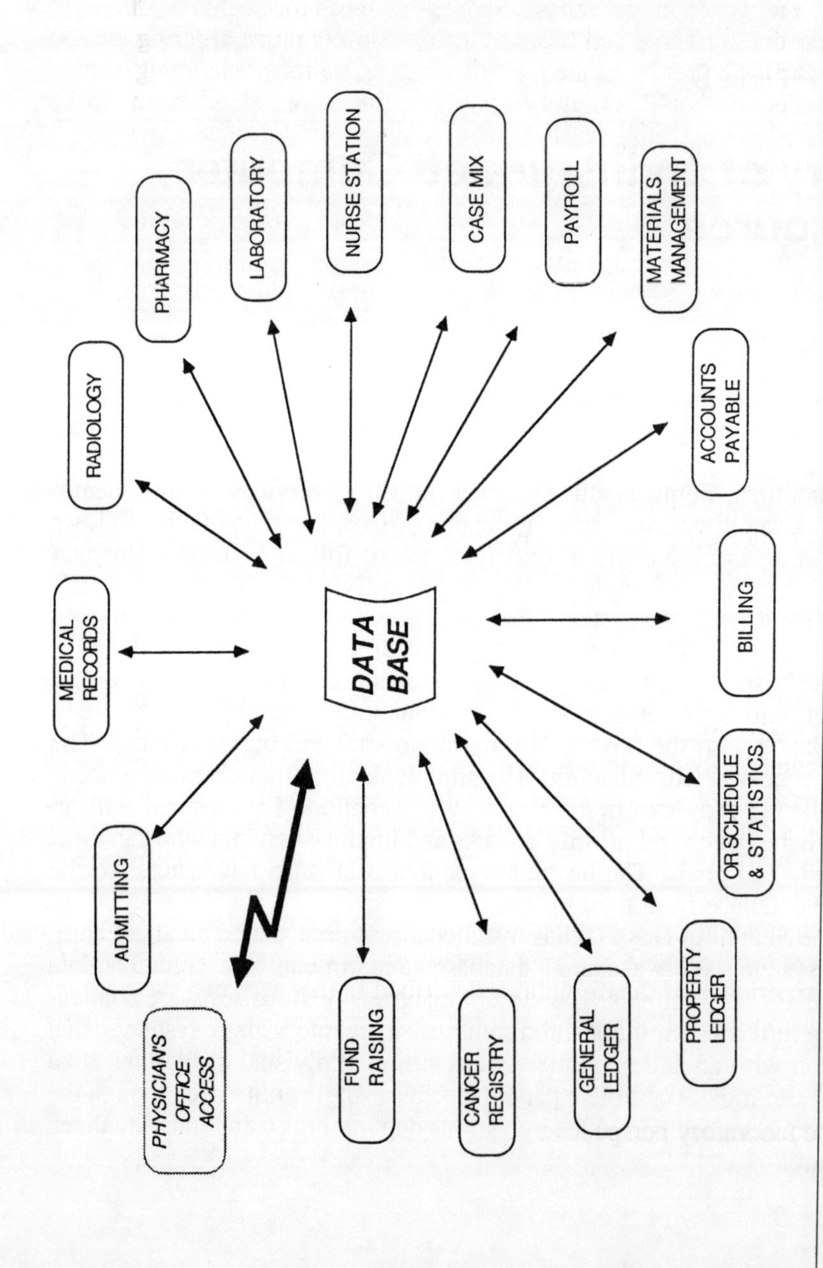

Figure 9-1. Shauntim hospital's real-time shared data base system. Reprinted from *The Health Care Supervisor*, Vol. 6, No. 3, April, 1988, p. 40, with permission of Aspen Publishers, Inc.

Among its various modules (Figure 9-1), the system includes the following: a registration and census module that feeds the shared database with patient demographic and location information; a nurse ordering and results reporting module located at all nursing stations, including the emergency department; a laboratory module with nearly all of its equipment feeding directly into the shared database; a pharmacy module that dispenses medications and maintains a patient medication profile; a radiology module that retains examination history and patient transcriptions; a case-mix module for the input of patient medical data and a report generator that provides analysis of data; and financial modules (the billing and accounts receivable module does the billing and collecting of patient charges as a byproduct of a service being performed).

The Integrated Approach: Planning and Compromise

Integration means hospital-wide real-time access to patient orders, test results, and demographic data. Integration has been difficult to achieve in most organizations because usually at least one department has selected, or wants to select, the optimal system for its particular needs even though such departmental needs may not always facilitate hospital-wide access. Integration means that each department compromises its specialized data needs and processes.

Optimizing each department's computer needs may not be in the best interest of the patient if hospital-wide access to each application's input and output features becomes impractical. Each support and ancillary department may need to compromise its specialized needs and features.

Today's solution is system-wide planning and preparation with compromise by individual departments and allied agencies. By using networked application languages and operating systems, Shauntim Hospital has been able to satisfy each department's major computer needs, while still being able to meet the hospital's overall patient information goals. The perspective and experience of the disciplines described in this scenario show the result of planning and compromise within one organization:

- the admissions and census perspective
- the laboratory perspective
- the radiology perspective
- the pharmacy perspective
- the nursing perspective

- the dietary perspective
- the physician perspective
- the physician's office perspective
- the medical records (case-mix) perspective
- the financial perspective

The Computer Steering Committee

The selection of Shauntim's system demanded input from all allied disciplines. The approach (Figure 9-2) was to form a steering committee composed of management personnel who represented their areas of responsibility and understood the system's goal of being driven by patient needs, not individual department needs. Trustees, physicians, nursing administrators, chief operating officers, chief financial officers, materials management managers, ancillary service administrators, consumers, and computer resource administrators made up the committee. As the selection process progressed, ad hoc members were invited to provide additional perspectives. The committee was guided by an outside consultant, with the hospital's central CR staff conducting the interviews, coordinating site visits and meetings, preparing the request for proposal (RFP), and analyzing the vendor responses.

Computers help meet information needs. Rather than ask each department what it wanted in terms of computerization, the staff designed a survey form that asked three things: (1) What are the information needs of the department? (2) How are these needs currently met? (3) What are the problems in meeting these needs? It took four steps to complete the needs survey:

1. The CR staff explained the form at a group meeting of department heads and supervisors.
2. The CR staff met individually with each department and reviewed its completed survey.
3. The CR staff responded to each department with the CR perception of the survey, suggesting ways in which the computer could be used.
4. The departments responded to the CR perceptions with additions and corrections.

Figure 9-2. The approach.

1. Define information needs and problems
2. Identify unique computer modules
3. Apply economic and patient care criteria
4. Prioritize modules
5. Prepare request for proposal for top priorities
6. Evaluate responses of vendors
7. Perform site visits and obtain references
8. Select vendors

The defined problems and solutions were then analyzed by the central CR staff. What at first was perceived as 50 different information modules was refined to 15. The 15 modules had to be prioritized because 15 was too large a number to handle at once. Each member of the committee prioritized each application in terms of perceived impact on patient care and system economics. Finally, the committee members met and, using their combined average as a guideline, reduced the priority list to six modules: medical records, registration and admitting, radiology, pharmacy, laboratory, and nurse station orders and results. The priorities of the remaining modules shown in Figure 9-1 would be determined at a later date after the first six modules were implemented.

A RFP that detailed the needs of each module and the format in which the vendors were to respond was prepared. Before it was sent to prospective vendors, the RFP was reviewed and approved by the committee.

Vendor responses were subject to various screening parameters; the major considerations are the factors shown in Figure 9-3. In addition, each proposed module was subject to intense review with site visits by the committee and appropriate users.

Modules

The registration and census module (admitting) and the medical records module provide patient data used by the nursing, laboratory, pharmacy, radiology, case-mix/medical records, and financial modules for patient-specific data and location. The modules make patient scheduling, preregistration, and registration efficient by retrieving stored patient data collected during the previous visit. On return visits, the patient is only asked questions particular to that visit. Before automation, each patient visit included asking

Figure 9-3. Selection criteria.

- System Flexibility
  - Previously installed (turnkey)
  - In-house or vendor software changes
- Availability of Applications
  - Medical record data and inpatient/outpatient registration/census
  - Order entry and results reporting
  - Laboratory
  - Pharmacy
  - Radiology
- Adequacy
- Growth Potential
- Hardware standardization
- Risk
- Cost

the patient to provide the same information provided on previous visits (i.e., date of birth, financial data, address, etc.).

The nursing module uses much of the data collected by the registration module and provides nursing with direct access for the ordering of ancillary tests. The previous manual ordering process required the use of handwritten and stamped requisitions that served as order forms, reporting forms for selected tests, and charge tickets.

The automated laboratory module uses patient data from the shared database and receives orders directly from the nurse station real-time module. When an order is placed via a VDT at the nurse station, it is automatically fed into the laboratory module. The laboratory module can handle the order on a routine, urgent, future, or STAT (at once) basis. Orders are printed on a collection list with labels. The results can be reported int three ways: (1) at the nurse station VDT; (2) through STAT broadcasting (automatic printing of results at a patient location when results are verified for release); and (3) via ward reports printed twice a day. Cumulative reports for patients' charts are provided once each day.

The pharmacy module, as with the other modules, requires its own unique data as well as data from the shared database. It automatically checks for drug interactions, indicates the amount to dispense, adds the patient's order to the profile and subsequent refill lists (if appropriate), produces labels, adjusts the inventory, and calculates and captures the correct charge. The patient medication profile is accessible at all nursing stations.

The radiology module retrieves any examination information entered during previous encounters, accepts orders directly from the nursing module and prompts entry for outpatient orders, and prints file room and patient control forms and flasher cards. The word processing feature enables transcribers to enter examination results quickly, as well as to insert coded comments. Eligible users with an appropriate confidential password can view current and historical patient profiles at any VDT. Charges are automatically sent to the financial module.

Currently, over 125 physicians have a password to access all the data. In addition, all features of the system are readily accessible at off-site physician offices.

The system has a case-mix module, which allows abstracting of selected data from the patient record to provide internal and outside agencies with hospital-specific data. The case-mix module is also used to monitor in-house patients by the utilization review staff. A major role of the case-mix module is its reporting capabilities; it allows the medical records department and the administration to create reports using data collected and stored in the shared database. The billing and accounts receivable module accepts data from the other modules in order to do third party billing and accounts receivable.

Quantifiable Benefits

There have been many quantifiable benefits from the integration of these modules. The results are getting to the medical staff faster, more completely, and more accurately. In the following sections, these varied benefits are discussed from many perspectives, including those of the physician, the nurse, the admitting officer, the radiologist, the dietitian, the pharmacist, the laboratory and medical records staff, and the financial officer.

Admission and Census Perspective

The admissions module plays a vital role in the shared and real-time database. Admissions is the site of the patient's first contact with the hospital, and there nearly all of the patient's demographic data are collected. These data will serve as the basis for nursing, laboratory, radiology, pharmacy, case mix, and finance modules and will not have to be reentered. The admissions module also provides standard question formats to ensure that clerks conform to the various and changing requirements of federal and state regulators and insurance carriers. The admissions module also serves as the control over patient location.

Inpatient and ambulatory preadmission scheduling and testing are important parts of the admission process. The shared database system ensures compliance with the regulations. The preadmission scheduling routines allow the admitting office to ensure complete and accurate demographic and insurance data, thereby making certain that patients meet requirements set by their insurance carriers.

The admissions module has been helpful in monitoring preadmission testing requirements for the patient who needs such tests and procedures. Nursing evaluations, anesthesiology assessment, and signatures must be completed before the scheduled admission date. Abnormal test results are known immediately, and additional or repeat procedures can be performed or admission can be canceled. The admissions staff has access to the laboratory and radiology modules to determine whether the proper process is followed and whether the appropriate tests are complete and valid.

Before the advent of a shared database, the ancillary department was called if the results were not sent within a reasonable period. Now the ancillary department no longer needs to send the information as data can be accessed by appropriate admission staff, thereby saving time. The ability of ancillary services to input and store test and procedure results allows designated personnel and physicians to view those results at a terminal and print them if needed. This accessibility saves numerous phone calls and saves time previously spent waiting for the results via interoffice mail.

The process of retrieving patient census by floor has opened communication between nursing units and the admissions office and is an important function in bed placement for incoming admissions and transfers. Nursing supervisors routinely use census reports to review occupancy concerns and to place patients.

Because patient information is stored real-time and is available 24 hours a day, a patient's medical records can be retrieved and reviewed before his or her impending arrival in the emergency department. Thus, if an ambulance calls with an expected patient the medical record can be retrieved quickly, before the patient's arrival. The automated system reduces search time, reduces patient waiting time, and provides accurate data and increased consumer satisfaction.

The admissions office makes use of the ability to send and receive messages wherever VDT and printer are located. Nursing sends messages directly to admitting to provide notice of pending discharge or transfer. At other times, a message is sent to all nursing stations when beds are short to ask them to respond with the number of upcoming available beds. The message system documents requests and notices that will often be forgotten in a busy admitting office dealing with the telephone. Thus, the system acts as the admitting offices' "memory bank."

Another major use of the message routine is its utilization by the short-stay registrar and the operating-room booking secretary. Staff in these two areas frequently leave messages in their respective "automated mailboxes" for such items as cancellations or emergency bookings taken late at night. Previously, they sent each other notes via interoffice mail if telephone contact failed. Now the use of both the telephone and interoffice mail is nearly eliminated.

The admissions module has allowed the department to maintain productivity while the workload has increased, without an accompanying increase in staff. Patients are processed into the hospital faster and with fewer errors than under the previous manual method. The ability to view laboratory and radiology data has made admission easier to perform and ensures compliance with physician and insurance-carrier requirements. Increased productivity and consumer satisfaction are the cornerstones of the shared real-time database, and it is vital to all departments and allied agencies.

Laboratory Perspective

Within a formerly totally manual laboratory, Shauntim Hospital computerized hematology, chemistry, bacteriology, urinalysis, radioimmunoassay, and serology. The change produced many benefits:

- Direct entry of results is possible by interfacing laboratory equipment with the hospital computer.
- Computer-generated labels make specimen labeling quicker and labels easier to read.
- Documentation of specimen collection time, the collector, and the time of receipt in the laboratory makes location, processing, and identification of specimens more efficient.
- Worksheets are prepared by the computer.
- The computer automatically captures charges and College of American Pathologists workload units and prepares management reports that are more detailed than could be obtained manually.
- Reporting of results is the biggest and most obvious benefit—results are now turned around faster, are more complete, are easier to read, and are in a real-time, retrievable format.

The laboratory currently has six pieces of laboratory equipment interfaced directly to the shared database. Three analyzers (two Coulter counters and an Astra-8) automatically enter hematology and chemistry results into the computer without operator transcription. This innovation greatly reduces transcription errors and incomplete results and saves technologist time.

Although the urinalysis section is not directly interfaced, it uses a digitizer pad to input results directly into the computer. This approach saves the technologist time because it greatly reduces the amount of time spent at a keyboard. (without the digitizer, it would be necessary to input "NEG" with four strokes on the keyboard, but with the digitizer only one key stroke is necessary). The hematology section also uses a coded keyboard for WBC differentials. The coded keyboard allows a technologist to utilize a standard VDT as a counting device. When the count is done, the results are already in the system, thereby eliminating the transcription step.

The laboratory has a bidirectional interface to the chemistry analyzer. The laboratory module transmits a list of specimens and tests to be run on the analyzer, eliminating many operator inputs. The operator runs the tests and transmits the results back to the laboratory module. This method reduces tedious results transcriptions, significantly reduces transcription errors, increases the completeness of results, and saves staff time.

Utilization of a computerized archival system makes data retrieval very easy. Patient laboratory results are available on the system after discharge/service for two years. After two years, the data can be retrieved real-time, but the data processing department has to make the file available.

Under the previous manual system, retrieval of old results was very time-consuming. A caller looking for test results needed to have the approximate date of service. The laboratory clerk would then search through carbon copies of the reports or through logbooks.

Changing a normal range is very efficient with the real-time system. Before the installation of the system, normal values were preprinted on the results forms. Whenever a change was needed, the forms vendor had to be contacted and asked to revise the form. This process took time and was very costly because of form set-up costs.

With the use of the computer, the presentation of patient laboratory results is far better than under the old manual system. Reports are more legible, correctly collated, and properly interpreted using normal and panic ranges, which are very age- and sex-specific.

Certainly, what has been gained by computerization can be gained from several good stand-alone laboratory systems. However, the hospital gained more benefits because the laboratory system is part of an integrated real-time database system. The system interfaces with all segments of the integrated systems. The admitting system automatically communicates to the laboratory all pertinent patient data. The order entry system allows the nursing staff to enter laboratory test orders, specify collection times and priority (routine, urgent, STAT, future), and note other pertinent information. From the laboratory viewpoint, orders are more specific (i.e., vague orders such as liver function tests are not possible), and the orders can be organized onto collection labels prepared in floor sequence by the computer. Result inquiry from the nursing station means that the nursing staff and physicians can view laboratory results. Previously, numerous telephone calls were received from staff looking for these results. Result inquiry has resulted in an immediate and dramatic decrease in the number of telephone calls into the laboratory and has greatly reduced the number of phone reports and associated errors. The STAT broadcasting system automatically sends STAT and urgent results to the patient location printer (even to temporary locations such as the recovery room) immediately after the laboratory technologist verifies the results. This method eliminates the need for laboratory staff to telephone inpatient and emergency department STAT results.

Laboratory charges are automatically captured by the computer when tests are requisitioned. Patient charges are virtually invisible to the laboratory staff. The computer eliminates the need to collect and prepare charge cards to send to data entry and eliminates the accompanying data processing calls for illegible and incomplete cards. Furthermore, the billing office does not call looking for missing laboratory charges because the system virtually ensures that all charges are accurately processed.

Another advantage of laboratory automation is report distribution. Patient test results are no longer hand-sorted from various laboratory sections. The daily chart copy for all results is printed by patient location for easy and fast distribution. Interestingly, chart copies have become less important as physicians use the VDTs for results. The VDT results can be viewed in chronological order in the same format as the chart copy.

Ultimately, even though the laboratory had to make some compromises on what capabilities were picked, the end result was a much more complete system. Another system that would make the laboratory even more efficient may have been selected, but it would not have been a system that easily fit into an integrated shared database. The ability to have result inquiry at any station and at the physicians' offices makes the integrated approach fit the laboratory's goal of providing accurate and fast results to the nursing and medical staffs.

Radiology Perspective

The radiology department has received many benefits from the shared computer system. Not only does the department have its own routines, but it also has access to data from other departments, such as registration and laboratory. Likewise, selected routines in the radiology system are used by other departments and the medical staff.

The radiology department has very successfully integrated automation into its daily operation. With the previous manual system, patients had to be registered in the radiology area, flash cards hand-typed, and orders provided on forms that were frequently illegible and incomplete. Indeed, time was frequently spent interpreting the language of the request or making telephone calls to the floors or physicians' offices to make sure that the proper test was performed. In addition, film jackets had to be located by referencing a large Rolodex file for the jacket number. The jacket number sometimes could not be located, and another number and subsequent folder would have to be issued. Thus, the ability to locate the old films was lost. File cards for the Rolodex had to be updated by hand with the examination name (it was updated if time permitted), or a new card had to be created with the patient demographic data and appropriate radiology data. Since the installation of the automated system, this Rolodex system has been eliminated entirely.

In addition to providing access to the film jacket number, the computer provides access to a patient's previous examination history at any terminal and offers easy reference for all persons in need of such data. Now a radiologist can quickly determine whether previous films exist and whether the jacket needs to be pulled for comparative films.

For each patient, radiology previously had to prepare a charge card and provide proper charge control documents before all papers were sent to data processing. Like other departments, radiology frequently received calls from billing or data processing if the charge data were incomplete or missing. Previously, all transcriptions were typed by hand. The turnaround time for results, if not STAT, would be 24 hours.

The automated and integrated radiology system has saved the hospital 2.5 full-time equivalents (FTEs) in the radiology reception area alone. This savings was attributed to a redefinition of the receptionist's duties as well as the elimination of patient registration in the radiology area. Necessary patient registration data (i.e., name, age, etc.) are now received as a by-product of the registration function. The radiology staff no longer has to type any documents. The computer printer provides all necessary documents using data already in the shared database. In addition, the preparation of file cards has been entirely eliminated as the computer maintains a history file of all examinations performed on the patient (maintained forever, unless the hospital chooses to delete patients not seen within the last five years).

When the receptionist enters the appropriate orders into the computer, a 3" × 8" form is printed and serves as the flash card, file room locater, and technician control. This form contains data from the shared database (i.e., date of birth, orders, clinical data, date of last radiology exam at the hospital, radiology file number, etc.).

The nursing staff uses its module to order radiology examinations directly from the nursing station and emergency department. The nursing order routine prompts the user to answer questions appropriate for each examination. Radiology now receives complete and legible information from nursing. Previously, radiology received handwritten order sheets that used terms different from radiology jargon. The order sheets were often incomplete, illegible, and late because they were hand-carried. Previously, nursing staff, in addition to writing the form, telephoned the order to radiology for clarification and scheduling. Telephone calls have essentially been eliminated, again saving staff time for both the nursing and the radiclogy departments.

The reception staff was previously responsible for preparing the charge cards. This step required a great deal of discussion with the technicians, and the charge cards were completely handwritten. Because charging is a by-product of the examination, this task has been entirely eliminated, saving both reception and technician time and forms.

The instant availability of the patient's radiology folder number increased the ability of file room personnel to locate jackets. With the latest date available, radiology staff knows whether to locate the films in the file room or in the five-day active file. The system also assists the file room in purging outdated folders and folders of deceased persons by identifying those patients not seen in five years or known to be dead.

The module allows the technologist immediate viewing, updating, altering, and correcting of examinations. Examinations may differ from what was ordered because radiologists have tailored the examination to the individual patient. This change is important both for professional accuracy and for proper and accurate billing. Previously, the completeness of the history of examinations was always subject to question.

Direct nursing order entry has increased the efficiency of both the nursing staff and the radiology department. The proper examination can be entered with the appropriate priority. Both the examination and the priority can be altered as necessary. The main benefit to the department is a decrease in the number of telephone calls and thus a decrease in noise pollution (with the elimination of more than 200 calls per day).

The system has a word processing capability for direct entry of radiologist dictation into the computer. Radiology can use a coding feature of the system to enter normal results in a standard format; the radiologist simply provides the proper codes and dictates additional information only if needed. The word processing and coding features have saved time for both radiologists and stenographers. Radiology, short-staffed in stenography, recently experienced a 20% increase in workload and would not have been able to survive without the system's word processing feature.

In addition, the transcribed results are available real-time for 60 days after the report. The reports are typed into the VDT and become available almost immediately to every nursing station, the emergency department, and many of the physicians' private offices. This availability decreases the number of telephone calls for reports and the time spent looking for old reports. Furthermore, this feature is used intensively by the clinical physician who, while making ward rounds, can immediately access the imaging reports and alter the patient's management accordingly. Similarly, the physician can dial into the reports from his or her office and have immediate access to all inpatient and outpatient imaging reports for the patient office visit. Direct access to reports by users has reduced time on the telephone for radiologists, receptionists, and stenographers.

The fact that the system is integrated allows the radiologist or the department of radiology nurse to access vital laboratory and pharmaceutical data on all of the scheduled special procedures and invasive examinations. Many of the procedures done in radiology use hepatotoxic and renotoxic materials, so it is necessary to see the latest kidney and liver laboratory tests; because the tests are invasive, radiology staff must know the results of all of the patient's significant hematological studies. In addition, radiology must know the history of an allergy and what drugs the patient is taking, as radiology patients are frequently medicated. The department does not want to use any drug that a patient cannot tolerate or any drug that will interact with a drug that the patient is already taking. Also, the contrast material used in myelography is contraindicated when phenothiazine drugs are being administered to these patients.

Special areas of importance for the chief of radiology are statistics on number and type of examinations being performed by shift, week, month, and year. Such statistics enable the chief of radiology to plan technical and professional staffing and also the purchasing, repairing, and updating of equipment. Statistics also enable the chief to advise the medical staff and the administration of any trends in examination (e.g., the marked increase in mammography that necessitated the establishment of a whole new program).

The radiology module has allowed the department to maintain a very efficient system in the wake of increased service needs despite no increase in staff. Furthermore, the radiology department has increased its ability to access accurate and complete patient data as it treats the patient and reviews prior films.

Pharmacy Perspective

As a result of computerization, the pharmacy department has experienced internal changes that have improved the quality and expanded the scope of pharmacy services. Before computerization, it was necessary for the pharmacists to maintain a handwritten drug profile for each patient in the hospital. With each new drug order, the pharmacist would retrieve the profile, enter the new orders, check for interactions or duplications, record the amount dispensed, and manually type a label for the initial doses to be sent to the nursing unit. If the patient's drug orders included intravenous (IV) medications, the pharmacist would enter the order into an additional profile and manually type individual labels for each of the IV bottles needed for each day's scheduled doses. At five- to seven-day intervals, each profile was copied so that medications already dispensed could be billed. A new sheet would then be typed to record future dispensings.

The billing of a patient for dispensed medications involved a technician using the profile and manually counting doses dispensed, looking up the current price of each drug in a price catalog, and extending the price with the use of a calculator. The billing paperwork was then batched and forwarded to the data processing department for batch entry.

The pharmacy department depended heavily on verbal and written communications for updating patient admissions, discharges, and transfers. If this information was not timely or accurate, medications might be sent to the wrong nursing unit or charged to the wrong patient.

After implementation of the pharmacy module, drug dispensing and record keeping proved to be far more efficient than manually maintaining profiles. With each order entered, the computer builds on the patient's previous drug profile and automatically checks each new entry for preprogrammed drug interactions or duplications. If duplications or interactions are found, the pharmacist is alerted. The computer calculates the correct number of doses to dispense and, if appropriate, the administration times and the order stop date. When the order is complete, the drug charges are automatically calculated based on up-to-date pricing. Simultaneously, the appropriate labels, for either unit dose medications or IV solutions, are neatly and quickly printed.

Considerable time was saved when the pharmacy module was first implemented merely because it offered a more efficient means of creating the patient drug profile and automated label printing and patient billing. However, the standard of pharmacy practice at Shauntim was more affected by computerization. Because of computerization, pharmacists no longer have to rely *solely* upon their own knowledge of drugs and drug interactions to be alerted to potential medication problems. Using the computer, the pharmacist can review in minutes the complete drug history of a patient or the complete dispensing history of a specific drug order when a question arises as to previous drug therapy. Consequently, the pharmacist now does a much better job interpreting drug therapy and identifying potential problems than was possible in the past.

In the IV area, the pharmacist is able to standardize the compounding of IV solutions because the computer provides an immediately available reference for mixing IV medications. In addition, because each medication dispensation is transacted via the pharmacy module, the overall documentation of drug dispensing has improved dramatically and, as a result, there have been parallel improvements in the accuracy and timeliness of billings.

The computer system has made it possible to store thousands of detailed discharged patient profiles on microfiche. These profiles can be kept in a desk drawer and are as accessible as the nearest microfiche reader. Previously, this same information was maintained as handwritten profiles and charge documents that created tremendous storage and information access problems. In the future, the pharmacy plans to eliminate the microfiche and to maintain discharge profiles with archival real-time storage.

In addition to the immediate changes to distribution functions within the pharmacy brought about by computerization, a number of changes in the scope of operations have been aided or made possible because of the pharmacy module's role in the hospital-wide database.

Shortly after implementation of the computer system, a satellite pharmacy was opened on the second floor of the hospital. From this satellite, the pharmacist can enter orders and distribute initial doses of medication and be readily accessible to medical and nursing staff for questions and reference. Previously, such medical and nursing staff contact had been limited. From the satellite pharmacy, the pharmacist also can print labels in the main pharmacy for drugs not available in the satellite and for IV medications compounded in the IV admixture area.

Because pharmacy is an integral part of the shared database, automatic updates on patient admissions, discharges, and transfers within the hospital are possible. Also, when drug therapies are monitored, patient-specific information important to pharmacy (such as height, weight, drug allergies, and primary diagnosis), which under a manual system was often incomplete or lost in the paper shuffle, now immediately appears in the pharmacy module when entered into other computer modules.

Finally, the ability to retrieve patient laboratory results in the pharmacy has also been a benefit of the shared database. The interface with laboratory, for example, has made it possible to review electrolytes and blood glucose levels in patients receiving total parenteral nutrients (TPNs) and to review bacteriology cultures and sensitivities of patients receiving antibiotics. Before installation of the computer, the review of laboratory results within the pharmacy was essentially impossible. In Shauntim's facility, the pharmacist utilizes the computer for concurrent and retrospective drug monitoring and utilization review operations, tasks that were literally unmanageable when the system relied on manually maintained patient profiles. Finally, in the administrative area, pharmacy has utilized the database management abilities of the computer to gain some independence from the accounting department in managing the drug budget and monitoring drug usage and pharmacy workloads.

Clearly, computerization has had its greatest impact on pharmacy as a profession, by automating and standardizing the more routine and traditional functions of the pharmacy (i.e., distribution and documentation). The pharmacist can now better utilize his or her training in more clinically oriented responsibilities.

Nursing Perspective

Before the implementation of the nurse order and results reporting module, the nursing units processed physician orders through a combination of activities. These activities included using the telephone, completing charge cards and department requisitions, delivering the charge cards and requisitions (by hand carrying or sending through the hospital mail system to the designated department), and transcribing orders to the nursing cardex. This process caused many problems: busy telephone lines, requisitions delivered to wrong departments (necessitating rerouting), and illegible penmanship. The audit trail for many orders reflected poor documentation of the actions taken.

Some departments used the original charge card as the results-reporting form that was returned to the unit to file in the patient's record. The interval of time between the ordering of the test and the return of the report to the unit was frequently filled with questions about the status of the test or result. If a physician or nurse wanted to obtain test results, the department had to be called and the results requested. Along with tying up the telephone lines, such inquiries caused frustration and frequent interruptions of work routines in both nursing and ancillary departments.

The order entry and results-reporting system has been operational with some departments for as long as two years. In spite of expected resistance to any new system, nursing is now in a position to appreciate more fully the benefits of the automation process:

- standardization of part of the process of transcribing physician orders
- reduction of error based on illegibility
- improvement in audit trail
- reduction of time between action on initial order and results availability
- decrease in duplication of tests
- improved access to test results

The nursing module has been designed so that one ordering screen is used for all orders. This design decreases the need for a user to learn different ordering methods. The unit clerk or nurse directly enters the physician's order request into the VDT. The patient's name or unique hospital identification number is entered, and the system automatically supplied the demographic data. The clerk need only read the line of information to confirm that the correct patient has been identified. Each ancillary department is identified by a mnemonic that historically was the department's nickname. Tests or examinations are entered one at a time using the test mnemonic, and the clerk proceeds through the screen formats answering examination-specific questions. Various prompts appear on the screen to remind the user that, when ordering a specific examination, some other action must be initiated. These prompt reminders decrease the number of incomplete examination preparations.

When the clerk schedules a test using a priority of routine, urgent, STAT (at once), or future, the physicians and all departments have already agreed on the word definition. Because of the standardized word usage, misconceptions and the need for corrections are eliminated, and time is saved.

All orders are entered into the system and immediately transmitted to the printer in the designated ancillary department. The format of the order output is standardized, legible, and timely and provides the department with unique patient data needs. With the faster and more complete orders, the ancillary departments are better able to arrange their work schedules.

Laboratory orders automatically print on a phlebotomy drawing list along with specimen labels. Phlebotomists, twice a day, deliver results reports to the nursing units. These reports list the tests of the patients who had laboratory activity that day, the tests' statuses, and results. The cumulative summary report is delivered early each day to be the chart copy of the patient's test results. These report forms are printed on 8.5" × 11" paper, which allows for easy placement in the records, data identification, and retrieval.

Another positive aspect of the system is that an authorized individual can use any VDT to view the status of a patient's tests; telephone calls for inquiry are eliminated. The user just enters a password and identifies the patient; the status and results appear. The user can see whether the blood specimen has been received into the laboratory, whether the test is completed, or whether results have been verified. In radiology, the user can learn that the roentgenogram has been taken, but the report is in draft form.

Results inquiry has greatly reduced frequent interruptions of nursing by physicians and residents. Shauntim Hospital has a residency program with Medical University in medicine, surgery, and pediatrics, and residents are performing patient rounds 24 hours a day. The medical and surgical residents now sit at the VDTs and view all of their patients' reports (with occasional reminding to vacate the terminal).

A feature termed Daily Profile has significantly reduced the duplication of test requests. The Daily Profile can be viewed on the VDT for specific dates. Nursing uses the printed profile as its "check sheet;" the evening clerk views what was ordered by the day clerk, thereby preventing duplication. In those instances of patients transferring to another unit, a printed Daily Profile becomes a quick and accurate means of one nurse reporting to another what was ordered and scheduled for that patient.

Another positive aspect of the system is that the time spent between nursing and an ancillary department is now quality time. Both departments are no longer burdened by a high level of frustration; open lines of communication exist and issues are addressed more quickly.

Entry of patient conditions has been made faster with the VDT. Previously, sheets were filled out twice a day for all patients; now, only the exceptions are entered into the system. The information desk views the condition and any appropriate restrictions or comments for that patient placed by nursing.

Dietary orders are also entered into the system. Previously, the patient diet type was handwritten on a sheet for all patients. Now, like patient conditions, only exceptions are entered into the VDT.

The module has a message capability; nursing can immediately notify dietary of any changes. In addition, the dietary department is automatically notified of admissions and discharges, resulting in a marked reduction in the delivery of meals for patients no longer on the floor and in calls to bring meals for new patients.

The message module is also used to notify admitting of pending discharges and other messages. Nursing also communicates drug changes and other pharmacy communications. Radiology uses the message feature to send STAT readings to the floors and to the emergency department. Before the message feature was installed, telephone calls and interoffice mail were used.

Dietary Perspective

The dietary department does not input patient or dietary data into the integrated systems, but instead makes extensive use of the access capabilities of the existing clinical and demographic data that other users enter. The computer has made possible the elimination of much of the hand-carried paperwork and the visits once necessary for communication between nursing units and the diet office.

The registered dietitians have patient information available at their fingertips to assist them in nutritional assessment and follow-up of patients. Clinical and pharmacy data are quickly accessed via VDT and aid in nutritional assessment and follow-up. For example, the albumin test might be looked at to find out whether a tube feeding was sufficient to replenish protein stores; a gallbladder scan might be viewed to see whether a change in diet would be necessary; medications would be scanned to determine whether elevated blood sugars were the result of a special medication or the nutritional feeding.

Previous to the integrated system and VDT access, the dietitian had to go to the nursing floor to review the patient record. The record was not available if the patient was off the floor or if the nurse or physician was using the chart. Inquiry into the patient record via VDT saves valuable dietitian hours and provides concise, accurate information.

Access to demographic data such as patient height, weight, age, and diagnosis allows dietitians to set priorities for patient care by diagnosis and nutritional status. For confidentiality reasons, all of this information is viewed by eligible users only.

The cardexes need to be updated three times a day to reflect all diet changes, new orders, or NPO orders for surgery or tests that have been made throughout the hospital. In the past, each nursing unit wrote all changes, and diet aides collected these handwritten sheets three times a day. Now the floors are able to update all diets before each meal via VDT, and the current lists are printed in the diet office and transcribed to the diet records. These lists provide information on patient locations, diets, tube feedings, food allergies, special needs, and precautions. In the near future, the cardex will be automated.

Information is also generated on the total number of meals served, with a breakdown for each specific diet category. This capability is helpful for budgeting and planning purposes.

All tray requests, new admissions, diet changes, and special meal requests are relayed to the diet office through the printer or as a message on the VDT. In addition, discharges and transfers are sent to the printer automatically as they occur throughout the day, allowing continual updating of cardexes. This updating saves many telephone calls and provides a record of communication. In addition, the message and notification capability of the system has reduced significantly the number of meals wasted because of patient discharges or delivery to the wrong floor. This is reflected in both work hour and material savings.

In the past, all patient menus for breakfast, lunch, and dinner were printed by hand with the patient's name, room, and diet. The computer now generates and prints labels, a tremendous saving of time. The time saved for the dietitians and diet aides by the integrated computer system is now used for greater patient contact.

Physician Perspective

It is impossible to appreciate the advantages of the computer-generated order entry and reporting system without reviewing what the organization was like before the system was implemented. In former times, an order for a laboratory test was set in motion by a ward clerk who would choose (from the many forms) the proper laboratory order form, stamp an addressed plate on the sheet, and make check marks opposite the requested tests. If the test was needed immediately, a call went out to a phlebotomist, who would pick up the slip just before drawing the specimen from the patient. In the past, a slightly misplaced check mark meant a wrong test.

Now, the clerk orders on a computer terminal from a menu of mnemonics that appear one at a time and that represent the actual name of the test. The clerk can add pertinent comments, if necessary. Mistakes, although they do occur, are less likely; the screen will show the retrieved order, and any necessary correction is only a few key strokes away. What's the difference? For one thing, time. Routine or urgent orders need a lead time of only about a half hour to be included in the next routine rounds. STATS still require a telephone call to request the immediate presence of the technician, but the required test requisition is already in the laboratory. Much of this takes place without the physician being aware of it, but the outcome is evident: more timely laboratory results.

There is obviously more to the order entry and reporting system. The test must still be performed, confirmed, and reported back. This has already been alluded to, but one aspect has proven critical. In the past, the physician, eagerly awaiting a result to determine the next step with a stick patient, would call the laboratory and eventually be put in touch with a technician in the right section, who would then determine the status of the test. If the test was completed, results might be retrieved by looking them up in a handwritten laboratory book. This process took the time of several people, including the physician, and often led to frustration when results could not be found. Now, the physician merely sits down at a terminal and calls up the results. If the results are not on the screen, they are not yet ready; if they have been verified, they flash before the physician instantly. If the test was ordered STAT or urgent, the results are printed on the patient's floor the instant they are available.

An additional benefit comes from the reporting medium itself. Results are not recopied from laboratory book to form, as previously, but often are generated directly from machine to computer. Transcription errors are markedly reduced. Formerly, the laboratory reports were on multiple small slips pasted side by side and often pasted incorrectly—even upside-down or sideways. These forms had a tendency, over time, to fall out of the stored record because the glue dried out, and they were often difficult to read because results were handwritten. Now, all laboratory results are printed on full sheets, are more easily read, and are correctly collated with previous results for easy review.

There is no question that this new system has produced a revolutionary change in patient care—so much so that physicians are even more impatient for results, even though they know that it would be difficult to make results appear any faster. The remarkable makes the impossible seem within reach.

The results of the system in radiology have been just as dramatic. The production of radiology requisitions was only slightly different from that already described for the clinical laboratory. Again, the possibility of error in ordering was greater with the written slips than it is now. The computer-generated order, again, appears in hard copy in the radiology department immediately after it is completed on the floor, and proper scheduling can take place quickly. The results of the procedure are no longer recorded at a typewriter but on a computer terminal directly into memory. Results in memory are available on screen the second the transcriber has finished entering them. This process avoids the telephone calls and waiting that once accompanied the process of getting early radiology reports and, of course, the final copy is printed by computer and is ready for delivery promptly.

Most recently, one feature of the pharmacy system has become available to the medical staff on-line. The physician can now review his or her patient's medications in one integrated list rather than having to refer to the cardex (which is sometimes difficult to interpret) or, even worse, having to look at the medication sheets (which are often not available at the central nursing station). There is little question that the clinical computer system has contributed enormously to a faster and more accurate flow of information to the physician and, therefore, has markedly improved patient care.

Physician's Office Perspective

Physicians' offices often need a copy of the patient's most recent laboratory and radiology report. In the past, a physician would call the hospital medical record department, and a copy of the report would be put in the physician's hospital mailbox or would be picked up. With the real-time system, physicians use the office accounting system computer and its telecommunication software. A physician can connect to the hospital through a dedicated line or modem and can immediately print the patient's reports on the office printer. Time is saved by not having the physician's staff go to the hospital. The new process saves time for the hospital staff by not requesting reports from them and for the physician by making reports immediately available as he or she is seeing the patient.

The system can also check whether the patient has had previous roentgenography at the hospital—for example, a chest film within the previous year—thereby often eliminating the need to order another one. In the past, the physician would call the hospital, and the radiology staff would look up the request in their files while the physician waited on the telephone. Waiting on the telephone and having to call the hospital are eliminated. Time and money are saved for both the physician's and the hospital's staffs.

The system can also be used to schedule the patient at the hospital. The physician sends the patient to the hospital for laboratory and radiology examinations, and the physician's assistant or secretary simply goes into the system and enters a scheduling routine. The assistant orders the type of examination necessary and actually schedules the patient from his or her office. The patient can report directly to the ancillary department without having to stop at the registration area. The hospital likes the new process because it saves registration staff time and reduces telephone calls to the physician's office from patients who inadvertently have not been given instructions as to what examinations they were to have. Patients also exclaim the virtues of this faster registration process as they spend less time in the registration process.

Another benefit of direct communication is access to the hospital's patient demographic data. Previously, with a consult, the physician received a copy of the patient registration form and copied the patient's financial information from it. With the direct connection, that financial data can now be downloaded to the physician's own database, saving time and increasing accuracy. In addition, when wrong information is discovered, such as inaccurate insurance numbers, the physician can now look at the account in the hospital system and through its billing sources obtain access to the correct data. When physicians receive returned mail, they are able to utilize hospital billing techniques because the hospital receives the rejected addresses also and has sources that locate the correct address.

Some physicians also have microcomputers in their homes. They use a modem to access the hospital's computer via dedicated telephone lines set up by the hospital. The system is particularly helpful when physicians are providing coverage for other physicians. Upon receiving a call at home, a physician can go to the computer and view the patient's laboratory, radiology, and pharmacy profiles. Prior to using their own microcomputer, physicians had to go to the hospital or else depend on the person calling to describe the patient's examination and treatment history.

Medical Record (Case-Mix) Perspective

The medical record, finance, and administrative departments make extensive use of the shared database and case-mix module. The medical record department is responsible for the integrity of that data.

One major advantage of the case-mix module is the capability of the records and finance departments to generate user-defined reports on the inpatient and outpatient populations. The system can select and summarize data on each of 250 data elements. The reporting feature gives users the ability to identify and analyze inpatient data such as frequency of diagnosis, cost of services, and other parameters. Without the case-mix module and the shared database, reports could not be provided with the level of detail and timeliness requested.

Previously, a paper abstract was prepared to collect demographic and clinical data on all discharged patients, a time-consuming and costly manual process. The completed abstract was forwarded to a data service that manipulated the information into a variety of standard indices and reports. The turnaround time was several weeks, and space was needed to store the reports. Requests for hospital-specific data not included in the standard output were obtained at additional cost, and lead time was needed to generate the information.

With the shared database, demographic information is passed over to medical records from admitting, eliminating repetitious entry and documentation. Verification and edit checks that are built into the system assist in maintaining the integrity of the data entered. All collected elements are stored for a specific period and are soon to be archived permanently to disk in a manner similar to the laboratory historical data. Once again, storage space requirements are greatly reduced.

Due to changes in the Medicare law, medical record departments are now an integral part of the billing process. The shared database allows coded data required by the billing office to be passed from medical records to the billing module. The diagnoses and operative codes are automatically grouped in the case-mix module, generating appropriate diagnosis-related group (DRG) data.

The utilization review function of the module allows concurrent monitoring of all hospitalized patients. DRGs are assigned on admission by the review coordinator and are appropriately changed during the hospital stay if the patient's clinical status changes.

The record department may receive copies of test results for discharged patients, and these results need to be put in the chart. Before the advent of the shared system, there was some difficulty in identifying the patient chart, for example, when only the patient name served as the identifier. Now each report shows a unique medical record number.

Laboratory reports are now printed in an efficient format. Previously, results were reported on cards that added to the record size.

The laboratory module is also being used. Third parties frequently request information regarding tests and dates performed. Before the shared system, the record would be pulled. Now the necessary laboratory data are simply viewed on the screen.

The medical record department benefits indirectly from the admission module. In the past, the emergency department would ask this department for patient telephone numbers and other necessary demographics so that they could contact the patient. Now emergency staff look up the data themselves, saving both medical record and emergency staff time.

In summary, the shared data system has enhanced the ability of the medical record department to respond to the increasing demands for complete and current data that reflect the use of hospital services.

Financial Perspective

The financial system receives most of the billing information automatically from the clinical modules. Patient charges for room, ancillary tests, and examinations are captured as a by-product of the service performed. Previously, each ancillary area prepared a charge card. The card was delivered to the data processing area and keyed into the computer via batch processing. This required staff time for ancillary data processing and handling. Furthermore, this process sometimes resulted in lost charges as cards were illegible or lost. The time between card preparation and delivery to the computer room could be as long as four days during a holiday period. In addition, late charges, charges applied to the patient bill after third-party billing, would have to be manually reviewed, prepared, and submitted by the billers. Depending on the amount, late charges might even have been absorbed by the hospital.

There is direct communication between the case-mix, medical records, and accounts receivable modules. The medical record department enters Medicare inpatient DRG data into the case-mix module. Medical record uses these DRG data when generating case-mix analysis reports, but the same data are also used to facilitate prompt billing of Medicare accounts. Previously, Medicare DRG data were telephoned to billing or sent via interoffice mail. This time-consuming process delayed billing. The present management report allows the billers quickly to recognize discharged Medicare accounts with no DRG.

Each biller has a VDT and can enter a patient's specific data into the computer. A complete account history is available immediately, and there is no longer a need to maintain a paper file folder for all accounts. Paper file folders and the handling and filing of various bills have been nearly eliminated, and only restricted accounts are maintained in a folder.

The accounts receivable system can extensively check patient data before the preparation of third-party bills. Billing clerks generate reports of errors by simply asking the computer to perform edit checks on accounts due for third-party billing. The clerks can then investigate such third-party errors as charges incompatible with diagnosis codes before the account is sent to the third party. The computer capability significantly reduces third-party rejections as billing errors are investigated and corrected before third-party submission.

The real-time access to all patient data allows the patient billers to handle telephone inquiries more efficiently. All telephone calls and other specific account inquiries and notes are recorded directly in the computer and can be referenced at any time. Thus, via the VDT, billers have access to such information as who took the patient call and what was the outcome. This real-time access has had a positive impact on the image of the hospital.

A report writer is available in the financial system, and eligible users have their own VDTs and enter and retrieve data on demand. A manager or supervisor can go immediately into the computer and prepare specific reports, such as aging by third party, and simultaneously monitor and develop methods better to manage receivable accounts. Before the integrated system, an analysis of the accounts receivable system had to be accomplished through separate programming requests that often, if data processing staff had time, took weeks. The integration of the financial and nursing systems played a major role in reducing the billing delay period from six days to four days. This decrease represents an additional cash flow for the hospital of $400,000. In addition, the data entry operation has been phased out because of automatic charging.

With an integrated system, patient bills are more accurate and timely. Charges are simply a by-product of the service performed. Users no longer must be monitored to make sure that they get their charges processed on time. The handling of late and missing charges has been significantly reduced. The reporting capability provides a means of reviewing and intensifying the analysis of accounts receivable.

Other Modules

In addition to the already-described system, literature articles address materials management, payroll, accounts payable, general ledger, property ledger, a regional cancer registry (O'Sullivan et al. 1981, Priest et al. 1980), and an operating room statistical and scheduling module (Priest et al. 1981).

A Key Ingredient for Success

Before actual implementation of the computer system, a user coordinator was appointed for each module. Figure 9-4 summarizes the responsibilities of the central computer resource manager (CCRM) and the user computer resource managers (UCRMs).

There must be one user coordinator for each module. This person must have an attitude of "It's up to me to make this successful." The UCRM does not necessarily have to have a computer background, but must have the initiative to learn and look beyond what is currently in place.

The coordinator must have the authority to make decisions regarding procedures, software, and hardware. This authority cannot be overemphasized. Many times a person has the capability to make decisions, but is not given the authority; unnecessary referrals to committees and departmental red tape can often hamper and delay an installation.

This UCRM must maintain communications in the department and with other users and serve as the expert on the module. He or she will be responsible for training the staff and must be familiar with documentation.

The computer resource (CR) staff members also play a vital role. CR staff members provide the main perspective on the integrated software and shared data and must be aware of all user needs, problems, and concerns.

Figure 9-4. The key ingredients to success.

THE SUCCESSFUL USER COMPUTER RESOURCE MANAGER

1. Is a member of the user staff
2. Has an "it's up to me to make this successful" attitude
3. Has the authority to make decisions/changes
4. Maintains communications among users
5. Is a documentation-type person: knows that the written word is a commitment; ensures that all areas are covered; assigns responsibility; communicates to all concerned
6. Uses CR staff members as a sounding board

THE SUCCESSFUL COMPUTER RESOURCE STAFF

1. Lets user coordinate/lead project
2. Is ready to take over the project if the user is not capable
3. Ensures hardware and computer access
4. Documents and communicates progress
5. Provides a perspective of the integrated applications
6. Monitors computer resources—space/response times/security
7. Chairs the "Work Committee"
8. Provides the systems perspective, i.e., flow, staffing, procedure changes, etc.

They must document and communicate progress to all users and to all levels of management.

CR staff members monitor the hardware and ensure that allotted space, response times, and security of hardware, software, and data are appropriate. They should chair the work committee of user coordinators that meets routinely to discuss progress, updates, and concerns.

The CR staff provides the system's perspective for patient and data entry flow, integrity of data, staffing, and procedure changes. The CR staff can be invaluable in assisting the UCRMs with their planning and systems techniques.

The CR staff must be prepared to take over the project if there is no appropriate coordinator or to realize when the coordinator is not handling the responsibilities. However, this move must be a last resort. It is critical to have a UCRM.

In summary, the success, failure, or delays of the system correlate directly with the effort and responsibility assumed by the user coordinators. In addition, the CR staff must provide the needed support for the coordinators to perform their job.

Table 9-1. CR Cost Indicators

Cost Indicator	Year 1	Year 2	Year 3	Year 4
CR $/Adj. Patient Days	$3.81	$4.94	$6.23	$7.54
% CR $/Operating Income	0.89%	1.0%	1.1%	1.1%
% CR $/Expenses	1.06%	1.2%	1.5%	1.7%

Cost Summary

The cost of purchasing and maintaining the hospital's computer resources can be expressed in various ways as summarized in Table 9-1. These CR costs include those in the CR budget (e.g., wages, supplies, maintenance for hardware and software) and hardware and software depreciation. The cost indicators do not include hospital overhead.

The hospital went live with its first real-time module in April. Over a three-year period, it implemented 15 modules (as shown in Figure 9-1). The current CR costs per adjusted patient day (inpatient days were adjusted by the percentage of outpatient revenue) is $7.74. Another CR cost indicator is that computer resource costs represent 1.1% of the hospital's total operating income and 1.7% of the hospital's total expenses.

Merely looking at CR cost indicators does not determine whether the hospital is getting the proper return for its investment. The hospital has reviewed published indicators (Dorenfest 1985) however, and it is certainly well within expected cost ranges. Indeed, given that the organization has acceptable CR costs and is satisfied with the CR services, the institution is indeed getting a good return for its CR investment.

Conclusion

This discussion has described the benefits to users of the selected modules of an integrated real-time shared database system (Figure 9-5). This scenario is meant to give one perspective on how ideas discussed in this text can be carried out in a real-world situation. Rather than using the fictitious Shauntim Hospital, we could have described the approach of steering committee, needs definition, vendor selection, and implementation in a nursing home, a home health agency, or another type of healthcare

Figure 9-5. Benefits of a hospital-wide shared database system.

- Physician
  - — Decrease turnaround time for test results
  - — Provide more patient and test information in a concise and legible manner
  - — Decrease number of patient and test data errors
  - — Provide complete patient data as a single entity

- Registration and Medical Record
  - — Reduce registration time
  - — Reduce number of registration forms
  - — Reduce patient data errors by recalling previous visit demographic data
  - — Eliminate storage for unit number recall
  - — Provide faster recall of patient demographic data
  - — Notify appropriate areas of patient location
  - — Improve communications with nursing and ancillary areas
  - — Provide access to result inquiry and improve preregistration and scheduling procedures

- Nursing
  - — Provide complete patient data as single entity
  - — Minimize duplication of orders
  - — Minimize lost orders and results
  - — Minimize incomplete test orders and results
  - — Reduce telephone calls among nursing stations and ancillary departments
  - — Redistribute nursing duties
  - — Improve timeliness, access, and accuracy of patient information throughout hospital
  - — Reduce duplicate paper files and transcriptions
  - — Reduce wasted meals and raw food inventory
  - — Eliminate trips by nursing aides to ancillary departments to deliver requisitions
  - — Eliminate manual retrieval of medical record to insert late test results
  - — Eliminate manually prepared midnight census, dietary, category of care, and condition reports
  - — Notify concerned areas upon patient order
  - — Eliminate charge ticket requisition forms
  - — Generate standard nursing orders
  - — Reduce size of patient medical record through more concise reports
  - — Improve communication with admitting through messages

Figure 9-5, continued.

* Pharmacy
  — Reduce drug inventory
  — Decrease medication errors
  — Eliminate manual pricing, typing of labels, and maintenance of patient profiles

* Laboratory
  — Improve test turnaround time
  — Decrease number of errors on what has been ordered and who receives test (test request more complete with appropriate patient information)
  — Decrease telephone calls from nursing stations and physicians
  — Decrease duplicate test requests
  — Provide easier test report to read with histologic test reporting, normals, abnormals, and deltas
  — Eliminate manually written results (increases result accuracy and legibility)
  — Eliminate manual pricing of tests

* Radiology
  — Facilitate faster access to films
  — Facilitate faster preparation of transcriptions
  — Provide access to laboratory results
  — Eliminate storage unit for film number retrieval
  — Provide real-time film history
  — Eliminate manual pricing of tests
  — Facilitate faster processing of patient through department

* Financial
  — Eliminate lost patient charges
  — Reduce billing lag days
  — Provide real-time access to patient billing information
  — Speed-up third-party billing process
  — Minimize late charges
  — Improve communications with medical record department for billing data

facility. However, the truth of the late 1980s is that only hospitals have aggressively attempted the breadth of computer resources and approaches described here. If one follows the definition, selection, implementation, and continual planning and monitoring process discussed, these concepts are appropriate for any type of health-care facility.

State-of-the-art computer technology will continue to change the way each health care facility functions. It certainly has standardized the manner in which the disciplines communicate. An integrated system, no matter which type of health-care facility in which it resides, can have a positive impact on the quality of patient care by providing timely, accurate, and complete patient data in an efficient and cost-effective manner.

Suggested Readings

Dorenfest, S.I. 1985. *The State of the Art in Hospital Information Systems*. Northbrook, IL: Dorenfest and Associates.

O'Sullivan, V.J., H.W. Neitlich, and S.L. Priest. Development of a regional computerized cancer registry and impact on medical care, in *Proceedings of a joint conference of the Society for Computer Medicine and the Society for Advanced Medical Systems*. Washington, D.C., October 30-November 1981, 10–12.

Priest, S.L., P. Arena, R.M. Cadieux, et al. March and July 1988. Implementation and application of a hospital-wide computer system. *Healthcare Supervisor* 6(3) and 6(4).

Priest, S.L., R.E. Clive and H.W. Neitlich. January 1978. Various experts work to shape computerized tumor registry. *Hospitals* 52(2): 69–72.

Priest, S.L., B.A. Pelati, and D.E. Marcello. June 1, 1980. Various experts work to shape computerized operating room log. *Hospitals* 54(11): 79–82.

Priest, S.L., B.A. Pelati, and D.E. Marcello. October 1981. A computerized operating room log and data base. *Journal of the Operating Room Research Institute* 1(5): 19–27.

CHAPTER 10

A Microcomputer Policy

Introduction

All chapters of this book have referred to microcomputers and their importance to the individual user and have discussed the microcomputer and its relationship to the organization. The following is given as one example of how an organization might present its microcomputer policy. The policy must recognize the scope of support provided within the organization. For example, an organization with a computer resources support staff (as discussed in Chapter 7) will have a policy philosophy different from that of an organization of limited budget and staff where users assume more of the support functions. All organizations that use microcomputers must address the microcomputer issue for management reasons discussed throughout this text (Hewson 1987; Walters 1987).

The Microcomputer Policy

Introduction

With the advent of the microcomputer, there is a need to develop policies and guidelines for the use and acquisition of microcomputers. The intent of a microcomputer policy is not to tie the hands of the user, but to provide management guidelines and support for growth and development both in the organization and in the end-user area. This policy establishes justification for a microcomputer policy, discusses when exceptions are permissible and the management responsibilities of such, explains the criteria used to select the specific hardware and software, and discusses microcomputer management issues.

General Policy

1. The purchasing staff is responsible for the acquisition of all microcomputer software and hardware.

2. The computer resource support staff is available to assist users in evaluation and selection of hardware and software, installation and trouble-shooting, and in training.
3. User personnel are not permitted to copy any licensed or copyrighted software programs onto any microcomputer. Proprietary software programs that are not licensed to the organization may not be executed on its microcomputers.

Exception to the Policy

Sometimes an application not supported inhouse may have to be run on a specific microcomputer not supported by the staff. In this case, the user must acknowledge that the advantages listed under the "Justification for Standardizing Microcomputer Types and Applications" may not apply to them.

Definitions

For the purpose of this policy the following definitions will apply:

Microcomputer. A microcomputer is a computer system that:

- is of desktop size
- including all hardware and software, can be purchased for under $15,000
- can be installed by the user or computer resource support staff with no ongoing hardware or software support, other than regular maintenance, required from the vendor

Hardware. Hardware is any piece or collection of physical pieces of electrical, mechanical, or electronic equipment that make up a computer system, including printers, visual display terminals, printer ribbons, diskettes, and the central processing unit.

Software. Software is any computer logic instructions or programs that will operate a given microcomputer system. There are several categories of microcomputer software:

- The operating software or system is the control programs that provide the overall function and operation of the microcomputer.

For example, the operating system can control where data are stored on a disk and how to reference the data.

- The application software is for specific user needs. Examples of this software are spreadsheet, graphics, and word processing.
- Custom software are programs written by the user to be used for specific applications and in one of the languages supported by the microcomputer.

Justification for Standardizing Microcomputer Types and Applications

There are many good microcomputers available today. Some are less costly than others. Others offer unique advantages for doing specific tasks. In any case, there are at least seven good reasons why this organization has limited the number of brands of microcomputers and accompanying software applications that will be supported.

Hardware Backup. If one's microcomputer is broken, there will be similar brands elsewhere to allow users to run backup diskettes and tape cartridges. Peripherals, such as printers, can be shared and interchanged.

Staff Backup. Staff in the same or another area will be familiar with how an application works and how the microcomputer operates. They can assist each other in learning the system and in training new users. The organization will not be disrupted because of staff inability to operate the microcomputer during illnesses, vacations, or terminations.

Software Portability. A software package developed or acquired by a user can be shared with others.

Host Communication and Report Downloading. A communication protocol can be established to ensure that there are no problems with microcomputers communicating with central computers.

Vendor Support. Buying in volume quantities gives better leverage for service, training, and pricing.

Computer Resource Staff Support. The computer resource (CR) staff can provide support and training to the user. With too many brands of microcomputers and applications, it is difficult for staff to acquire the necessary expertise.

Networking. Similar microcomputers and software offer present and future opportunity for microcomputers to talk to each other. Files can be easily downloaded and uploaded, and data can be shared.

Supported Hardware and Software

The microcomputer and application software listed were selected after comparing various packages considering their user-friendliness, recognition in local schools and colleges, the market share of each package, and the knowledge of a package by in-house staff:

Software

1. Word processing—Word A
2. Spreadsheet—Spread B
3. Graphics—Graph C
4. Database manager—Data D
5. Host communication and downloading—Comm E

Hardware

The microcomputer and printer were selected to support the software packages. All models of microcomputer brand ABC (X1, A2, P3) were used.

Printer Issues

The printer was selected based on the following criteria:

1. Most printers have their own unique ribbon. An unlimited number of printers means that there is a need to stock a multitude of ribbons.
2. One needs to be aware of staff and hardware backup. When users use the same printer, the staff will be familiar with its operation, such as how to change the ribbon, how to load paper, where to turn it on, etc. In addition, similar printers can be swapped without having to be concerned as to whether the printer is compatible with the microcomputer or software.

3. The repair of the printer is a factor. Where will the maintenance come from? If not in-house, is there a local firm that will support the printer? Do they have parts available? A printer with no available service can be a frustration to a user who must send it by express for repair.
4. Other factors were: speed of the printer ; physical size (where it will be located); dependability; quality of print (i.e., near letter quality versus letter quality); graphics capability; desktop publishing; paper size to be used (i.e., 8" × 11" and/or 11" × 15"); and price (which plays a role in all factors).

The following printers are supported locally and are compatible with the selected microcomputers and software.

- Printer 41—near letter quality—If absolute best quality is not necessary and you will not do desktop publishing, this is the chosen brand.
- Laser—publishing—Most expensive; justification must include a need for publication quality output.

Purchasing Support and Maintenance

The organization has a contract for repair of all microcomputer hardware and peripherals. If there is a need for hardware service, call the purchasing staff (X0009). They will obtain service and maintain a log of maintenance services.

Software Assistance

If there is a need to obtain assistance in using an application, or if there are perceived software bugs, the following steps should be taken:

1. Look at the reference manual. Does it explain your need?
2. Can another user supply support? Perhaps one of your fellow employees has experienced a similar problem.
3. Call the software's customer assistance number.
4. Last, call the Computer Resource Support staff.

Software Updates

As each software package is purchased, it is registered with the support vendor by the purchasing area in purchasing's name. As updates for the software are received, they are logged in by purchasing and distributed to the user areas. With this system, all areas will be using the same version of the software.

Microcomputer Management Issues

Each user who will manage a microcomputer must submit a plan addressing the following management issues:

1. Hardware security—How will you protect the microcomputer? Will it be by padlock, locked room, constant supervision? Microcomputers and their supplies (ribbons, paper) are expensive and subject to theft and vandalism.
2. Software security—How are the programs protected from unauthorized change?
3. System backup—Who is responsible for protecting the data via backup to diskette or tape? How often is it done? Does the person using the microcomputer know how to back it up?
4. Access/confidentiality—Who can use the computer? How is the data protected from unauthorized access—password and/or restricted access area?
5. Database integrity—Who updates the database? Are there regular checks made to ensure the accuracy and completeness of the data? Do you do duplicate entry at times to verify a certain percentage of accuracy?
6. File management—How often do you purge files? Who is authorized to purge files?
7. Space and capacity limitations—How much data can be stored? How is it monitored? How frequently? What happens if you go to file away data and there is not enough space?
8. Multiuser—If there are more than one user on the microcomputer, who is the master user? What about access to files by all users?

9. Network administration—Are the microcomputers that you want to use compatible with the network that they will be operating on?
10. Communications and compatibility—Do the microcomputer and software allow downloading and sharing of files? Are they compatible?
11. Accuracy—Are programs and formulas audited with test data to ensure that there are no logic and calculation errors? The test should include incorrect input data to see whether the system recognizes them. Accuracy tests include printing the formulas and having another person in the department verify them. In addition, reasonable tests can be made on the output information.
12. Documentation—Who will ensure proper documentation of how to use the system and its applications? Who is in charge of seeing the documentation updated with current changes and returned to its proper area? Documentation includes functional narratives, flow charts, and operational procedures.
13. Support—Do you know how to do first-line maintenance, i.e., change ribbons, switch lines, load paper, ensure that the terminal is turned on, etc.?
14. Backup plan—Does a backup plan exist that tells what to do when the microcomputer is not working? What happens when power is off? What happens if you lose data before you back up? What happens if there is an equipment failure?

Microcomputer Committee

A monthly meeting should be held of all microcomputer users. The purpose of the meeting is to share concepts and applications among the user community and to provide continuing microcomputer education and dialogue.

Suggested Readings

Austin, D.J. 1988. *Information systems for health services administration.* 3rd ed. Ann Arbor, MI: Health Administration Press.

Harris, W.L., Jr., and J.C. McAllister. December 1985. Microcomputer applications for home health–care services. *American Journal of Hospital Pharmacy* 42(12):2702–2708.

Hewson, T.S. June 1987. Managing the growth of microcomputers in healthcare. *Healthcare Financial Management* 68–72.

McClymonds, B., and P. Howard, June 1985. Evaluating the microcomputer-based cost system. *Computers in Healthcare* 18–24.

Schmitz, H.H. 1987. *Managing health care information resources*. Rockville, MD: Aspen Publications.

Walters, R.F. 1987. *Database principles for personal computers*. Englewood, NJ: Prentice–Hall.

CHAPTER 11

Implementing Tomorrow's Healthcare Computer Resource Network

Introduction

Tomorrow's healthcare computer network has each individual's medical history as the focal point, regardless of where the individual is physically located. A person's medical history will be as close to him or her as are the telephone and other communication devices. Access and updating of individual medical data will come from hospitals, extended care facilities, home health-care providers, physicians' offices, school systems, mental health agencies, satellite clinics, and other organizations with an interest in providing accessible individual care. Data will be shared among these various providers from a single database. Essentially, this database will contain each person's medical care history and will progress from prenatal life to death.

This scenario recognizes that the individual is the hub of the computer resource (CR) network (Figure 11-1). Each health-care provider accesses the centralized database of medical information to support its varying levels of activity. This includes referencing the history and past experiences of treatment and results. With the individual as the focus of the database, there is a need for each provider to share individual information with others.

The prenatal and birthing center will establish the person in the database; each individual's database will be expanded by ambulatory care providers, acute care hospital visits, physical therapy services, and other associated specialists. The database could even be accessed by early intervention school agencies. Eventually, the individual may be served in a long-term care facility or retirement (life care) community. He or she may receive home care. As the individual progresses through life, the frequency of access to the computer resource services will depend on that person's health and special needs.

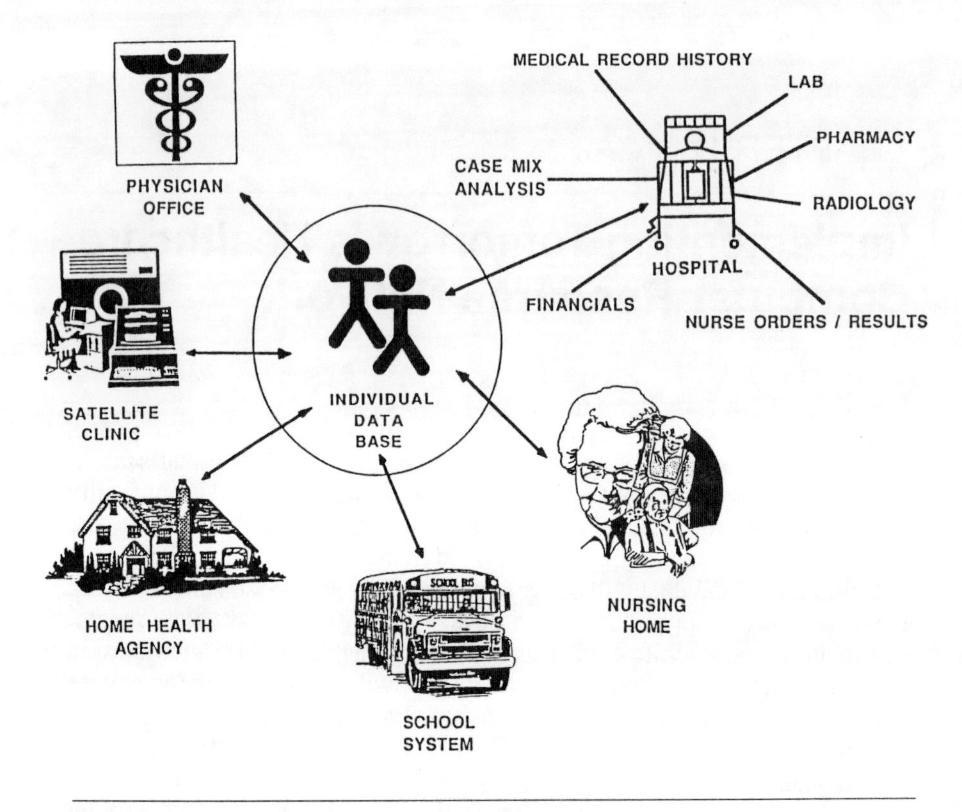

Figure 11-1. The Healthcare Computer Network.

The Holding Company

The financing of the computer resource network will be sizable. The CR network will most probably result because of mergers and acquisitions of provider organizations. Individual organizations within a holding company could include hospitals, extended care facilities, home health-care agencies, ancillary services such as laboratory and radiology, and even a real estate firm that services physician group practices. Outside organizations such as schools and nutrition programs will be allowed to access and update selected areas of the patient database. For example, a school might be allowed to access data on a student. A school nurse with a need to determine the number of diabetic students coming into the school during the next year will use the network to plan appropriate programs. Potential diabetic students will be identified by searching the database for individuals with a diabetic diagnosis, a certain zip code, and particular age range.

A nutrition agency will be able to scan a hospital's discharges for patients who will require home nutrition services. As the database expands, other social programs will also identify their potential population via the computer network. Restrictions and privacy protection policies will be strictly enforced and monitored.

A computer resource company will be part of the holding company and will offer an opportunity for a large degree of standardization of hardware and software. For instance, all organizations in the network will be required to use the same laboratory software. Standardization of software makes communication between different organizations less costly and more efficient to implement and maintain. Standardization will minimize the political red tape for departments and organizations having to select from a mixture of alternative software applications. Essentially the holding company will set the standards for hardware and software. Most organizations today have difficulty in getting agreement between users on which specific vendor and applications best meet their needs. This problem will not go away in the immediate future. The bias from previous experiences will be present when selecting vendors.

A holding company that mandates standardization of computer resources within its group of companies will minimize implementation and ongoing communication problems. The author believes that the holding company concept will be cost-effective and will provide adequate funding to maintain and enhance an integrated and up-to-date network.

The holding company will form a multidisciplinary steering committee using staff from within its member companies. It will go through an evaluation and selection process similar to what has previously been described. The steering committee will also serve as an ongoing group to monitor and promote the computer resource network. The evaluation of vendors and applications will be made in conjunction with the committee and the computer resource company. One criterion for selection insisted upon by the holding company will be that vendors must be able to both access and update the network. Another criterion will be that the individual must be the focal point of the system. Access to medical history and needed data must be maintained within the network.

The order in which individual organizations implement applications will be determined by each organization working with its own steering committee. An individual organization that wishes to deviate from the holding company's preferred software and hardware will have to demonstrate that communications and maintenance needs can be effectively met. Maximizing the efficiency of a given user or organization at the expense of the individual being the focal point of the network will not be permitted.

The network will never really be complete and, as new organizations join the holding company, outside agencies will recognize a need to access the medical data. National and regional legislation will address confidentiality and individual rights and needs, and the network must be able to adjust and change.

Technology is Not the Challenge

Computer resource technology in the 1980s is refined such that various types of hardware and software communicate with minimal technical problems. Optical disk technology uses a laser beam to update and store individual medical data for each visit within the network. Retrieval of specific vist data is immediate. However, the challenge of working with multiple vendors that offer different services and getting vendors to communicate with each other and develop schedules for the benefit of users is a management challenge.

Experience has shown that getting different vendors to work on an integrated system can pose problems. Such system integration needs as collecting patient demographic data using vendor A's registration and scheduling software and sharing the collected data with vendor B's laboratory software through the database of vendor C will be the management challenge of the computer network. Determining which vendor is responsible when the network does not work will be difficult. Which vendor changes to meet the specifications of the other? Which vendor is responsible for troubleshooting the problem when it seems that the problem could be within a multitude of areas? These will be the challenges of managing the computer resource network.

Hardware vendors present the same challenge. For example, a simple telecommunications system involves at least four areas, each of which may have a different vendor. The video display terminal is that of vendor 1, the modem transmission device is that of vendor 2, the telephone lines are leased from vendor 3, and the computer receiving the transmission is that of vendor 4.

A further major challenge exists when the organization choses to maintain the various applications on-site and each application is written in a different language, runs on a different computer, and uses a different operating system. The technology exists to meet the challenge, but the question is whether the organization's management can meet the challenge.

Thus, today's technology is not a problem. The problem and challenge will be getting various vendors with diverse interests, services, capabilities, and customer support philosophies to work together. Being able to select the most effective software and vendor for a particular user, such as laboratory, is certainly within the best interests of the laboratory and ultimately the organization and network. Being able to select the radiology software that meets the philosophy and needs of that area is in the best interest of the radiology staff. However, can vendors provide these applications and still be able to communicate effectively and meet the CR network demand for each individual's medical data?

The communication challenge of multiple vendors is solvable. However, it is difficult to coordinate and is a task that many organizations may not recognize until it is too late.

Confidentiality Versus Patient Health

The issue of access to private medical information is going to play a role in whether the computer network can be used to its fullest to provide individual health services. Legal concerns with protecting individual medical records will probably restrict the breadth of services and access. For example, the ability for all providers, worldwide, to access a person's record is well within the technology of today. However, the need to know will most likely restrict access to a regional area until audit trail and other confidentiality issues are legislated.

One method of protecting confidential medical data is for the data to reside in only two areas: (1) at the individual's last place of service and (2) on a wallet size card containing the identical medical history as the last place of service. To use the data on the card, an organization would place the card in a reader device and transfer the data to their local database. The card could be read by telecommunications devices such as those carried by an ambulance (Glaser 1988).

The Paperless Medical Record

Optical disk technology will be the medium for the paperless medical record. Figure 11-2 displays the manner in which a hospital would use this technology to store, retrieve, and ensure the completeness of individual medical data. The means of input into the database will be twofold: First is the usage of existing computer interfaces to pass data from one computer to another. For example, blood analyzers and roentgenograms will be passed from an organization-specific computer to the central database. Other automated input means will be the use of optical scanning and voice entry. The second method of input will be from direct entry via scanning paper documents. The individual's past and present medical history will be accessible throughout the network.

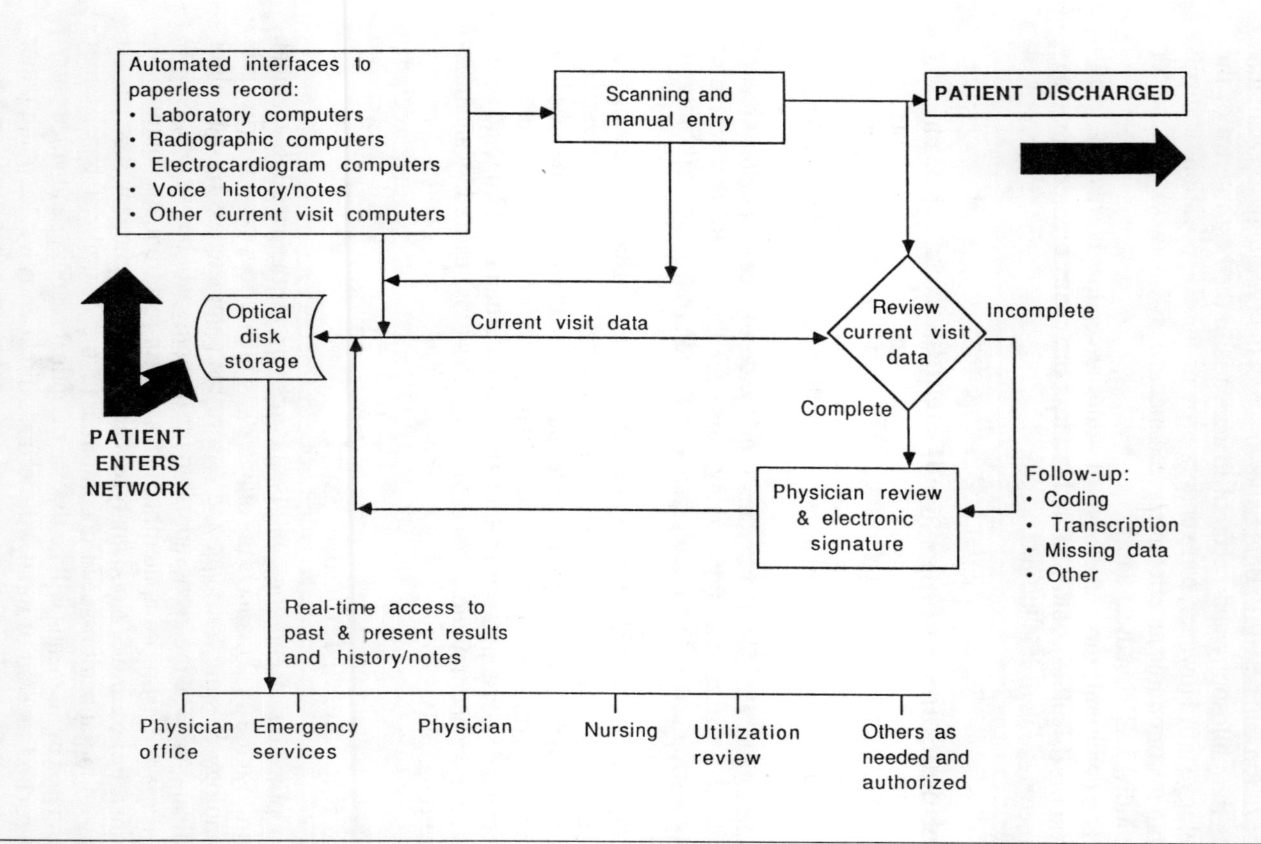

Figure 11-2. The paperless medical record.

The staff currently responsible for medical records storage and retrieval will find itself in the role of ensuring the completeness and integrity of the paperless medical record. It will further audit and ensure that access to the record is on a need-to-know basis.

Output will come in many forms. First is the visual screen, which will be able to display multiple windows of medical data on one screen and in color. For example, one will be able to view a roentgenogram while also hearing the radiologist's impression. Other results will be voice output for previously transcripted histories in current, summary, or detail sequence as determined by the operator.

Confidential data will be protected through voice recognition, handwriting analysis, palm recognition, genetic analysis, and other physical means. Electronic signatures will be analyzed. Another means of protecting data will be to have the central database dial back the calling computer and verify both user authorization and calling location.

Benefits for Users

Individuals

The individual is the foremost benefactor of the computer network. The person benefits in both cost and quality of care. When data are presented uniformly, physicians and other healthcare providers look at the same data. No matter how and when they were collected, the data are presented uniformly. A physician will see whether a test was given previously and will determine whether those results can be used now. This will mean fewer tests and less redundant data.

The computer network will also help analyze the data so that physicians all can start at the same beginning point. They can look at graphs and see changes more readily than when looking at a table of data. Trends will be recognized more easily and quickly. A faster interpretation of the data will occur with analytical tools such as graphs, which will allow the physician to focus on important details rather than trying to interpret raw data.

Data from previous diagnoses and results can be viewed graphically and compared to the present diagnosis and results. When changes in test results occur, the physician will be able to see the results more uniformly and completely. For example, laboratory results can be viewed concurrently with the effect of medications being taken to see the impact, if any, of the medication.

Another example is being able to view a bacteriology specimen while hearing the pathologist's interpretation at the same time. The same benefit is obtained with electrocardiograms and any other procedure where it is important for the physician to see the actual scan being interpreted by another physician. As the person goes from hospital to clinic to extended care facility, the data will automatically be available and used for current situations.

Hospitals

Faster, more complete, and more accurate results will be available to physicians and other hospital personnel. The presence of computers will be one measure of quality care.

There will be more efficient departmental operation through the monitoring of production and the retrieval of statistics. Most equipment will be connected to the central database, and there will be minimal manual input of results into the database. All equipment will be interfaced.

A paperless medical record will be possible. Optical disk technology will provide access to such data as on-line roentgenograms and electrocardiograms. Voice entry of nursing and physician notes and orders will significantly reduce medication and transcription errors. Access to these data will include computer voice response to requests.

Access to the patient's history will allow physicians to learn from the previous treatment of the patient. Suggestive diagnosis made using a universal database compared to each patient's particular symptoms and exam results will significantly impact diagnosis and reduce the length of hospital stay.

Bedside access to the patient's history and exam results will mean better continuity of patient data from previous treatments and diagnosis (Drazen and Huske 1988). Graphic output of results and monitoring criteria will reveal trends and other directions.

Patients will interact with computer-prepared television screens. Diet orders and training needs will become more personal for each patient.

Extended Care Facilities

Most of the benefits noted for hospitals will also be available at the extended care facility:

- Access to result data
- Paperless medical record
- Access to previous history

School Systems

Data to develop programs will be available.

Home Health Providers

- Statistics
- Access to previous history
- Increase in remote diagnosis at home via telecommunication and other devices interfaced directly with a medical facility and database and the patient at home
- Computer chips containing the individual's medical history will be implanted on the patient. Many diagnoses and treatments can be made at remote facilities while the patient remains at home. People with chronic problems such as diabetes will have their history immediately available to all healthcare providers with a need to know.

Nutrition Agencies

- Identification of hospital-discharged and home care patients requiring services
- Ability to plan meals based on previous diagnostic results

Physicians' Offices

- Access to previous history; servicing patients while they remain at home
- Orders placed to the hospital with identification via special passwords and identification devices (i.e., voice identification, eyeball identification, etc.)

Satellite Clinics

Satellite clinics will also have access to the previous history and other benefits.

Conclusion

This discussion has briefly shown issues that will be of vital concern in providing an individual healthcare computer network. The major problems will be legal questions and the coordination of multiple users. Technology will be available, but the restrictions placed on it by government, medical, and corporate politics will be more challenging than the technology itself. There will be a need for a myriad of organizations to work together. As long as the individual is the ultimate focus of the computer network, the system will grow and play a significant role in the cost and quality of medical care.

Suggested Readings

Carter, K. September 11, 1987. Hospitals taking lead in efforts to integrate information systems. *Modern Healthcare.*

Chambers, A.L. October-November 1987. Speech technology in the emergency room. *Speech Technology* 50.

Drazen, E., and M.S. Huske. 1988. Bedside terminals: Promises versus reality. *Topics In Health Records Management* 9(2): 18-25.

Glasser, J.P., N. Mann, and J. Edgar. 1988. Smart cards in health care: Current status and future prospects. *Topics in Health Records Management* 9(2): 26-35.

Goldberg, A.J., and P.F. Abrami. August 1988. *The technology interface: state of the art of nurse station bedside terminals.* Burlington, MA: Applied Management Systems, Inc.

Roland, J.C. October-November 1987. Voice technology moves in the nursing home industry. *Speech Technology* 34.

Sager, B.B. Fall 1988. Voice technology—is it ready? In *DATA*. Billerica, MA: Medical Systems Management, Inc.

Yankee Group. October 1988. *Survey: optical disk as a mass storage peripheral-mass storage management summary.* Boston, MA: Yankee Group.

Yankee Group. October 1988. *1987 end-user survey of the digital document and image automation market.* Boston, MA: Yankee Group.

APPENDIX

"My Entire Computer Files Have Been Destroyed!"

Introduction

This is a scenario that actually took place. The names and places have been changed to protect the guilty, but the facts are accurate. The scenario relates the sequence of events initiated when a physician responsible for his group practice's accounts receivable system called a consultant. The consultant was called because the physician had been told by the microcomputer vendor that the office's accounts receivable files were destroyed.

The scenario is presented as an example of what can happen when dependence on computer resources is not accompanied by knowledge of how to manage computer resources.

The Scenario

Shaun Timado, a computer consultant, received a call from Dr. John Smith, a local physician who was part of a group practice. Dr. Smith was very perplexed. He had just been told by his computer vendor that his computer files had been destroyed, no backup files existed, and he would need to reenter into the computer the entire accounts receivable file. This was both a monumental task and a questionable one because the thousands of accounts, with each account's detail, would first need to be located. The group's microcomputer disk was destroyed, and the backup diskettes were no good. The entire database was lost. Could the consultant help him?

It was clear that Dr. Smith did not quite understand what had happened. Mr. Timado called the vendor who had sold Dr. Smith the accounts receivable software and microcomputer, and the story unfolded: It had been a week since the Group's office manager had taken a job elsewhere. She had been the expert on the system, and the staff had turned to her when there had been a computer problem. The present staff was inexperienced on the system.

On Friday, the computer files were backed up in the morning per established procedures. On Sunday, an inexperienced clerk used the system and mistakenly put the system into a recovery mode, indicating to her that the backup files had to be loaded. She inserted the backup diskettes, but instead of updating the computer files she deleted the backup files from the diskettes. The system still indicated a recovery problem and the clerk did not know what to do, so she shut the system off and went home. On Monday, she did not tell the other member of the staff what happened. When the second inexperienced clerk started the system, she had the same message to load the backup files. She followed procedures that required using the oldest backup diskettes, but rather than restore the files, she did a format and deleted the last remaining set of backup files. After the diskettes were entered, the system again indicated recovery mode. She called the vendor representative who knew nothing of the aforementioned problems. He instructed her to follow the backup procedure using the second set of diskettes. The system message was "no data files existed." He then was told of the previous problems, but by this time the two sets of backups had been destroyed.

The vendor representative at first believed that recovery was impossible and that the entire accounts receivable and patient visit history files would have to be reentered using whatever source documents could be located. This was told to Dr. Smith, who of course could not believe that this disaster was happening. Visions of bankruptcy flashed through his head!

The vendor, however, was doing his best to determine how to recover from the backup diskettes. After intensive investigation, it was found that only the directory had been deleted from the diskettes. The data files still existed. Even so, it took two days of vendor programmer effort before the files were finally recovered. The files were restored to their condition after the last backup.

This still left the problem of catching up. Two days of data would have to be located and reentered. After much searching, the staff found the source documents from the two days before the disaster and reentered the data into the computer. In addition, the week's normal work was behind, and this had to be entered. Of course, while this was going on, no patient or insurance carrier bills could be mailed.

In summary, a disaster that happened in seconds required over a week for recovery to normal operations. This of course does not include the expense of overtime, lost revenue, frustration, worry, etc. How could one prevent this from happening again?

The Recommendations

The following recommendations for controlling the group's computer files were made:

1. Every day, at the end of the day, back up the computer's files onto one of five backup sets. Label each set as Monday, Tuesday, etc. If the office is open on weekends, have a set for Saturday and Sunday. On Friday, make a duplicate of the backup and remove it from the building. (This prevents loss in case of fire, theft, etc.) Permanently save the end-of-year and end-of-month backups.
2. All current staff should be trained by the vendor regarding accounts receivable (A/R) procedures and microcomputer operation. As new staff are hired, they should go through the same training sessions. All staff must know how to use the applications and operations manuals before they use the system.
3. At least two members of the staff should be cross-trained on the A/R and patient history applications. Previously, only one person had been trained on each application. With two cross-trained staff members, you will be able to have adequate coverage in case of vacations, sickness, terminations, etc.
4. The daily computer backup duties should also be rotated on a monthly basis.
5. There should be instructions describing the daily, weekly, and monthly procedures for the A/R and patient history applications and for the computer backup process. This will serve as a checklist to train new clerks and ensure that all procedures are carried out. The instructions should specify backup procedures and how to complete control logs to maintain file balances. The instructions should identify the specific reports used with the control logs to verify the system's master file totals.
6. All problems with the computer should be logged and reviewed daily by the office manager.
7. Source documents should be maintained and easily accessible for one week before being filed away or thrown out. If computer files are destroyed, the source documents will be used to reenter the data since the last backup. If the computer site is destroyed, the off-site backup is the only backup; therefore, one must maintain the source documents for at least one week.

Conclusion

Attention to proper management of one's computer resources is important. Microcomputers offer opportunities not possible when computer technology was managed solely by CR professionals. However, along with the opportunity provided by the new technology, there are additional responsibilities to manage them.

This scenario could happen to you!

Suggested Reading

Covvey, H.D., N.H. Craven, and N.H. McAlister. 1985. *Concepts and issues in health care computing*. Vol. 1. St. Louis: C.V. Mosby.

INDEX